THE TOP 100 HEALING FOODS

THE TOP 100 HEALING FOODS

PAULA BARTIMEUS

dbp

DUNCAN BAIRD PUBLISHERS

LONDON

THE TOP 100 HEALING FOODS

Paula Bartimeus

For Sri Chinmoy, my spiritual teacher who for many, many years has moulded and enriched my life beyond my imagination. Although he no longer resides on the earth plane, his presence is felt all-where and he shall eternally remain my inner and outer guide.

First published in the United Kingdom and Ireland in 2009 by Duncan Baird Publishers, an imprint of Watkins Publishing Limited, PO Box 883, Oxford, OX1 9PL

A member of Osprey Group
enquiries@dbp.co.uk

Managing Editor: Grace Cheetham
Editors: Ingrid Court-Jones and Amanda Hemmings
Managing Designer: Suzanne Tuhrim
Designer: Luana Gobbo
Commissioned photography: Simon Smith and Toby Scott

A CIP record for this book is available from the British Library

ISBN: 978-1-84483-758-8

10 9 8 7 6 5 4

Typeset in Helvetica Condensed
Colour reproduction by Colourscan, Singapore
Printed in China

Publisher's Note: The information in this book is not intended as a substitute for professional medical advice and treatment. If you are pregnant or breastfeeding or have any special dietary requirements, allergies or medical conditions, it is recommended that you consult a medical professional before following any of the information or recipes contained in this book. Duncan Baird Publishers, or any other persons who have been involved in working on this publication, cannot accept responsibility for any errors or omissions, inadvertent or not, that may be found in the recipes or text, nor for any problems that may arise as a result of preparing one of these recipes or following the advice contained in this work.

Notes on the recipes
Unless otherwise stated: • Use fresh herbs • Do not mix metric and imperial measurements
• 1 tsp = 5ml, 1 tbsp = 15ml, 1 cup = 250ml

Watkins Publishing is supporting the Woodland Trust, the UK's leading woodland conservation charity, by funding tree-planting initiatives and woodland maintenance.
www.dbp.co.uk

CONTENTS

KEY TO SYMBOLS

 anti-microbial

 anti-cancer

 anti-inflammatory

 antioxidant

 balances blood sugar

 detoxifying

 good for the heart

 good for the skin

 good for the brain

 helps the digestive system

immunity-boosting

introduction

"Let food be thy medicine and medicine be thy food."

HIPPOCRATES

Our ancestors knew well the healing power of natural foods and turned to them to combat all manner of maladies. It's only now, centuries later, that research has begun to confirm that the therapeutic benefits of these foods can be scientifically proven. In fact, some foods have been found to work even better than drugs – and without the adverse side effects.

From apples and almonds to honey and brown rice, this handbook will help you to get to know the many amazing medicinal properties found in everyday foods and learn which ones are useful for particular ailments. These top 100 healing foods not only prevent a wide range of health concerns but help to alleviate them as well. And note that nearly all these foods are available from your local supermarket or health food shop, apart from one or two ingredients which you may need to locate in a more specialist store. Mind you, you'll know they are worth finding when you realize the difference to your health – and hence to your life – such foods can make!

Most experts now agree that eating a diet rich in natural, health-giving foods can help us to ward off common complaints such as colds, coughs and infections as well as to protect ourselves against chronic degenerative diseases, including cancer, heart disease and arthritis. So, next time you're feeling below par, instead of turning to the medicine cabinet turn to your own fridge or kitchen cupboard where, with the help of this great book, you're likely to find a remedy.

To make the book easy to use, the carefully selected 100 wonderfoods have been divided into six main, colour-coded sections: Vegetables; Fruit; Grains, Beans and Pulses; Nuts and Seeds; Herbs and Spices; and Others, which includes an assortment of interesting food items. Each food entry offers practical and reliable information, along with a simple delicious recipe suggestion, a nutrient list and at-a-glance symbols highlighting its key healing properties. In addition, there are ten star foods that are specially highlighted for their remarkable health secrets and each of these includes two recipes. Finally, at the back of the book, you'll find an ailments directory for easy reference.

FOODS THAT HEAL
VEGETABLES
If there's one food group we can never eat too much of, it has to be vegetables. Abundant in vitamins, minerals, fibre and water, vegetables help to cleanse and alkalize the body, neutralizing acidity and reducing the toxic load. They are also low in fat and calories (with the exception of starchy vegetables, such as potatoes, eddoes, winter squash and yams) and are one of the best sources of phytochemicals – potent plant compounds that help to protect the body against disease.

Scientific research suggests that phytochemicals slow down the ageing process and reduce the risk of diseases and health concerns, including cancer, heart disease, high blood pressure, cataracts, osteoporosis and arthritis. Most of them function as antioxidants, helping to counteract the hazardous effects of free radicals – unstable molecules that damage body cells. In fact, free radical damage is thought to be one of the main causes of ageing. Phytochemicals exert various other mechanisms, such as stimulating the immune system, regulating hormones and providing anti-bacterial and anti-viral activity. The great news is that all vegetables are brimming with these natural plant components, of which hundreds have now been identified.

Try to make vegetables a central feature of main meals and find new ways of incorporating them into your diet, so that you eat generous amounts every day. When preparing salads, instead of sticking to basic ingredients like lettuce, cucumber, tomatoes and carrots, use them only as a base, and add a variety of other colourful ingredients such as celery, red pepper, radicchio, beetroot, fennel, watercress and mooli. Cooked vegetables are good too, especially in the winter. To preserve fragile nutrients such as vitamin C, steam, stir-fry or bake them rather than boil them, or add them to soups and stews. Juicing is another great way of reaping the goodness from vegetables in a more concentrated form.

FRUIT

Generally fruit contains more vitamins than vegetables, whereas vegetables rate higher in the mineral stakes. Most fruits are exceptionally cleansing and alkalizing, helping to eliminate toxins from the body and to regulate the digestive system by stimulating movement of the digestive tract and improving the body's ability to absorb nutrients. Fruits are also a fantastic source of enzymes, natural sugars and cell-protective phytochemicals.

As the body digests fruits relatively quickly (within 30 minutes), they are best eaten on their own, separately from other foods that take longer to digest. This prevents them from fermenting in the digestive tract. Between meals is probably a good time to fit them in, unless you opt for an all-fruit breakfast.

Both fresh and dried fruits are nutrient-rich, with dried fruits also being an excellent source of minerals. While freshly pressed fruit juices are good for you, it's advisable to dilute them with water to reduce their fruit-sugar content. This will help to curb blood sugar fluctuations and lower the calorie count, which can add up when fruits are juiced, as well as reduce the risk of dental caries.

STORE CUPBOARD TIPS

• Most vegetables should be stored in the fridge to help slow down their deterioration. It's best not to wash or chop them up until ready to use as they have a natural protective coating that helps to keep them fresh. Mushrooms are best stored refrigerated in paper bags. Don't refrigerate garlic, onions, winter squash and potatoes – they can be left uncovered in a cool dark place and eaten within a week or so.

• With the exception of berries, grapes, fresh figs, melons and pineapple, most fruit can be stored at room temperature until ripe. To speed up ripening, place fruit in a closed paper bag out of direct sunlight.

• Store grains, beans and pulses in airtight containers in a cupboard and label them with their use-by date. Once cooked, they will keep in the fridge for up to three days. Cooked beans can also be frozen.

• Unrefined vegetable oils are best kept in the fridge with the exception of olive oil, which solidifies unless kept at room temperature. Unrefined oils turn rancid quickly when exposed to heat and light.

• Nuts, seeds and their butters also contain oils and should be kept refrigerated to prevent them from going rancid.

• Fresh herbs can be preserved by placing their stems in small water-filled glass jars and covering them with clingfilm. They should then be refrigerated. Keep dried herbs and spices in clean, dry glass jars with airtight lids and store them away from light and heat to prevent loss of flavour.

GRAINS

Grains are the primary source of energy for many people throughout the world. Unrefined grains are rich in slow-releasing carbohydrates that help sustain and fuel the body. They are also rich in fibre to aid digestion.

There are two main types of fibre – soluble and insoluble. Soluble fibre helps to stabilize blood sugar levels and to lower high cholesterol, while insoluble fibre regulates bowel movements. Grains contain both types.

Some grains, such as quinoa and amaranth, provide the body with complete protein; other grains need to be combined with beans, pulses or seeds to make their protein more usable by the body. This can easily be achieved and we often do it automatically when preparing meals in traditional combinations –

for example, in beans on toast, rice and dhal, rice with chilli beans, and so on.

Like fruit and vegetables, grains have many healing vitamins, minerals and phytochemicals. Most grains supply B-vitamins, which are needed for normal metabolism and a healthy nervous system, along with calcium and magnesium and various trace elements.

If you are allergic or intolerant to gluten (a sticky protein found in wheat, rye, barley and oats), there are plenty of grains which are gluten-free, such as rice, millet, buckwheat, quinoa and amaranth.

BEANS AND PULSES

Collectively known as legumes, beans and pulses (the edible seeds of certain legumes) are an excellent source of protein (especially when combined with grains), as well as soluble and insoluble fibre and complex carbohydrates. This makes them ideal energy foods for balanced blood sugar. They also contain a broad spectrum of minerals and a brain nutrient called lecithin. If legumes cause you to bloat, their gassy effects can be avoided by adding a few bay leaves or a strip of kombu seaweed during the cooking process.

NUTS AND SEEDS

Both these food groups provide protein, minerals and vitamin E, which are very important for the skin, reproductive organs and circulatory system. They are also packed with the healthy fats associated with lowering high cholesterol, balancing hormones and reducing inflammation. The high fat content of nuts and seeds means they are calorie-laden, so eat them in moderation. They are ideal sprinkled on salads, cereals and desserts or as snacks. Also, nut and seed butters make tasty spreads on toast or crackers.

HERBS AND SPICES

Besides adding taste and aroma, herbs and spices boost the nutrient content of all kinds of meals. They also make fabulous substitutes for salt and some aid the digestive process.

To preserve the nutrients and flavour of both fresh and dried herbs, add them to dishes toward the end of the cooking time. However, it's best to add spices earlier to allow their flavour to develop fully. As well as being a real treat for our taste buds, herbs and spices can be made into medicinal teas (see box, above) to help to relieve various health problems.

HOW TO MAKE A MEDICINAL TEA

Place 50g/1¾oz fresh herbs or 1 heaped tablespoon dried herbs or spices in a saucepan, pour over 600ml/21fl oz/2⅓ cups of boiling water and cover. Leave to steep for 10–15 minutes, then strain. For coarser parts of the herb, such as stems, roots and barks or for spices, simmer the ingredients for 20 minutes to allow the goodness to be released. Infusions will last up to three days in the fridge and should be drunk two to three times a day.

OTHERS

There are some foods that do not fit into any of the categories mentioned so far, but without which no book on healing foods would be complete. These include protein-rich items, such as turkey, salmon, eggs and bio-yogurt; condiments, such as apple cider vinegar, which has long been valued as a curative; and natural sweeteners such as honey, carob, blackstrap molasses and xylitol. In some cases, such as dark chocolate, scientific research has only recently verified its array of healing benefits.

Additionally, a few Oriental treasures, such as miso, umeboshi plums and kuzu, have been included because of their exceptional medicinal and culinary uses.

USEFUL INFORMATION

• All recipes have been designed to serve four, although quantities may vary according to the size of the portion required.

• Always opt for organic food wherever possible. Organic produce is believed to contain more nutrients than intensively farmed food, and is free from potentially harmful chemicals.

• In an age when food allergies and intolerances are becoming increasingly prevalent, the saying "one man's meat is another man's poison" is absolutely accurate. So just because a particular food is endowed with therapeutic properties, do not assume that you will not react to it. Remember that it can still make you feel unwell if you are sensitive to it. If you suspect that you are reacting to certain foods, it is wise to get a comprehensive food allergy test.

Common food allergies include meat, fish, dairy, eggs, soya, wheat, gluten, nuts and yeast, although any food can be potentially problematic.

• Some healing foods possess naturally-occurring toxins, such as goitrogens and oxalic acid, which may aggravate specific health conditions. Fortunately, most of these compounds are deactivated during cooking. However, potatoes, tomatoes, aubergine and peppers contain substances called solanines that may exacerbate arthritis, as can citrus fruit.

cucumber

NUTRIENTS
Vitamins B3, B5, C, K, beta-carotene, biotin, folate; calcium, iodine, iron, magnesium, manganese, phosphorus, potassium, silica, zinc

The high water and mineral content of cucumber is largely responsible for its therapeutic cleansing and hydrating effects.

The expression "cool as a cucumber" is probably founded upon this vegetable's extremely high water content, which gives it refreshing and cooling qualities. Cucumber is a good source of the mineral silica, a component of connective tissue found in the skin. This, coupled with cucumber's large percentage of water, helps to keep skin cells well-nourished and hydrated. Cucumber can also be used topically to relieve various skin afflictions, including puffy eyes and sunburn. The vitamin C and caffeic acid in cucumber, which relieve inflammation and water retention, may explain why it is so effective for the skin.

GARDEN SALAD

100g/3½oz baby spinach leaves
1 cucumber, chopped
8 radishes, trimmed and thinly sliced
2 carrots, peeled and thinly sliced
1 spring onion, trimmed and chopped
2 tbsp chopped parsley
1 tbsp olive oil
juice of ½ lime

Combine the vegetables and parsley in a large bowl. Pour over the olive oil and lime juice, and toss well. Serve immediately.

tomato

Bursting with vitamin C, tomatoes are also packed with lycopene, one of the most potent cancer-fighting phytochemicals.

The exceptional feature of tomatoes is their high concentration of lycopene, a carotenoid compound which gives them their bright red colour. A higher intake of lycopene in the diet has been associated with a reduced risk of several cancers, including those of the prostate, lung and stomach. It has also been found to protect the skin from sun damage. Tomatoes are rich in potassium, which regulates fluid balance, and are an excellent source of vitamin C, which boosts the immune system.

NUTRIENTS
Vitamins B3, B5, B6, C, E, K, beta-carotene, biotin, folate; calcium, iodine, iron, magnesium, manganese, phosphorus, potassium, zinc; fibre

TOMATO RAITA

30 cherry tomatoes
400g/14oz/1⅔ cups bio-yogurt
1 spring onion, trimmed and finely chopped
1 tbsp finely chopped coriander leaves
1 tbsp finely chopped mint
½ tsp roasted ground cumin
sea salt to taste

Cut the tomatoes into quarters, place them in an oven-proof dish and grill until slightly soft. Leave to cool, then transfer to a bowl. Add the yogurt, spring onion, coriander, mint, cumin and salt. Mix well and serve as a dip.

Cooking tomatoes increases their lycopene availability and anti-cancer properties.

red pepper

NUTRIENTS
Vitamins B3, B6, C, E, K,
beta-carotene, biotin, folate;
calcium, iodine, iron, magnesium,
manganese, phosphorus,
potassium, zinc; fibre

RED PEPPER SAUCE

**2 red peppers, deseeded and
    chopped
250g/9oz cashew nuts
1 tsp freeze-dried dill
1 clove garlic
1 tbsp chopped onion
pinch of black pepper**

Put all the ingredients in a
food processor and blend until
creamy. Serve over grains or
steamed vegetables or use as
a sandwich spread.

The wide range of nutrients in this colourful vegetable
make it a great all-round immunity-booster.

Red peppers have a high water content, which helps to flush
out toxins from the body. They are also packed with vitamin C
and beta-carotene, useful for warding off colds and infections,
and fortifying the immune system. One 150g/5oz serving
contains an average person's daily needs of these vitamins.
Like tomatoes, red peppers are one of the few foods containing
lycopene, an antioxidant with anti-cancer properties.

004

fennel

This pale green bulb is packed with disease-preventing antioxidants and can be eaten either raw or cooked.

Fennel is a natural diuretic and promotes health in the liver, kidneys and spleen. Like many vegetables, it contains phytochemicals, including rutin, quercetin and kaempferol, which all act as powerful antioxidants. Rutin strengthens blood capillaries, thereby improving poor circulation, while quercetin inhibits inflammatory conditions such as asthma. Kaempferol has been found to reduce heart disease risk. Anethole, another compound in fennel, is anti-spasmodic, preventing the intestinal spasms often experienced by people with irritable bowel syndrome.

NUTRIENTS
Vitamins B3, B5, C, E, K, beta-carotene, biotin, folate; calcium, iodine, iron, magnesium, manganese, phosphorus, potassium, selenium, zinc; fibre

SAUTÉED FENNEL

1 tbsp olive oil
2 fennel bulbs, trimmed and
   finely sliced
8 cloves garlic
ground black pepper

Heat the oil in a pan, add the fennel and gently fry the garlic until slightly soft. Season with black pepper. Serve as an accompaniment or with some crusty wholegrain bread and cheese.

celery

NUTRIENTS
Vitamins B3, B5, C, E, K, biotin, folate; calcium, iodine, iron, magnesium, manganese, molybdenum, phosphorus, potassium, selenium, sodium, zinc; fibre

Containing concentrates of many amazing therapeutic compounds, just three celery sticks make up one of the five recommended daily portions of fruit and vegetables.

Vital minerals can be lost in the sweat following vigorous exercise or during a fever. Celery juice, with its high concentration of water, potassium and naturally-occurring sodium, can help to replace this loss by hydrating the body and restoring electrolyte balance. As celery juice has a strong flavour, it is best mixed with other juices, such as carrot.

Celery leaves can be trimmed off and used for flavouring soups and salads.

CLASSIC WALDORF SALAD

5 celery sticks, finely chopped
2 apples, chopped
medium bunch white seedless
** grapes**
1 spring onion, trimmed and
** chopped**
a handful chopped walnuts
2 tbsp mayonnaise
2 tbsp bio-yogurt
½ tsp celery seeds
ground black pepper to taste

Put the celery, apples, grapes, spring onion and walnuts in a large bowl. Put the remaining ingredients in a separate small bowl and stir well. Tip the mixture onto the salad and mix well. Serve immediately.

REDUCE STRESS EFFECTS

With its rich mineral content, celery helps to normalize the body's acid–alkaline balance. An acidic state caused by stress or eating harmful foods can lead to numerous health problems. Celery seems to counteract this acidity, thereby improving conditions such as fatigue, rheumatism and joint pain.

BLOOD PRESSURE BONUS

Besides being a natural diuretic, celery has been found to lower high blood pressure. Compounds called pthalides help to relax the muscles around arteries, allowing blood vessels to dilate. This provides more room for blood to flow, hence lowering the blood pressure. Other healing compounds in celery include coumarins, which enhance the immune system, as well as acetylenics, which have cancer-fighting properties.

CELERY WITH COTTAGE CHEESE AND CHIVES

6 celery sticks
250g/9oz/1 cup cottage cheese
a handful of chopped pecan nuts
1 tbsp finely chopped chives
ground black pepper to taste

Cut the celery sticks into generous bite-sized pieces. Mix the cottage cheese with the nuts, chives and pepper, and use it to fill the ribs in the celery sticks. Serve as a light lunch or snack.

leek

NUTRIENTS
Vitamins B1, B3, B5, B6, C, E, K, beta-carotene, biotin, folate; calcium, iodine, iron, magnesium, manganese, phosphorus, potassium, selenium, zinc; fibre

For low cholesterol and a super healthy heart, leeks should be included in the diet on a regular basis.

Leeks are related to garlic and onions, and contain many of the same health-promoting compounds as these vegetables. According to research, they lower total and LDL (bad) cholesterol, increase the HDL (good) cholesterol and bring down high blood pressure – making them a wonderfood for the heart and circulatory system. Regular consumption of leeks is also associated with a reduced risk of several forms of cancer, while their combination of vitamins and minerals helps to stabilize blood sugar levels.

LEEK AND PECAN SAUCE

1 tbsp olive oil
1 leek, trimmed and chopped
50g/1¾oz/½ cup pecan nuts
1 tsp ground mustard seeds
1 tsp wholegrain mustard
200ml/7fl oz/¾ cup milk or soya milk
1 heaped tsp dried thyme
½ tsp vegetable bouillon powder

Heat the oil in a pan and sauté the leek until soft. Then, place it in a food processor along with the remaining ingredients and blend until creamy. Serve either hot or cold on potatoes or other vegetables.

aubergine

This versatile vegetable protects the brain from ageing and may help to keep infections at bay.

Well-known as a main ingredient in the Greek dish moussaka, aubergines contain many beneficial substances including nasunin, an anthocyanin found to protect fats in brain cells from free-radical damage, which may help to slow down the ageing process of this vital organ. Another important healing compound found in aubergine is chlorogenic acid, whose potent anti-viral, anti-bacterial and anti-fungal properties are thought to aid the body in resisting infections.

NUTRIENTS

Vitamins B3, C, K, biotin, folate, beta-carotene; calcium, iodine, iron, magnesium, manganese, phosphorus, potassium, selenium, zinc; fibre

AUBERGINE GRATIN

2 aubergines
3 tbsp olive oil
100g/3½oz Cheddar cheese or
    dairy-free alternative

Cut the aubergine into slices and brush the sides with the oil. Arrange them in an oven-proof dish in overlapping slices, cover with foil and cook in a preheated oven at 220°C/425°F/Gas mark 7 for 25 minutes. Remove the foil and cook for a further 10 minutes. Take out of the oven, sprinkle with the grated cheese and place under a grill until the cheese has melted.

asparagus

High in nutrients, low in calories and rich in flavour, asparagus has many health benefits to offer.

Vitamins B1, B3, B5, C, E, K, beta-carotene, biotin, folate; calcium, iron, magnesium, manganese, phosphorus, potassium, selenium, zinc; fibre

According to folklore, asparagus is considered to be a tonic for the reproductive system. It's an excellent source of folic acid (which protects against neural tube birth defects), and beta-carotene and vitamin C – antioxidant nutrients which help to fight cancer, heart disease and eye problems. Asparagus also works as a mild diuretic, thanks to its high potassium content and asparagine, an amino acid found in this vegetable. Eating asparagus makes the urine smell in some people, but this effect is quite harmless.

Eat asparagus as soon as possible after purchasing, as it tends to toughen up quickly.

ASPARAGUS, EGG AND SWEET PEPPER SALAD

10 asparagus spears, chopped
1 red pepper, deseeded and thinly sliced
3 tbsp olive oil
3 hard-boiled free-range eggs, shelled and chopped
2 tbsp chopped chives
2 tbsp chopped parsley
ground black pepper

Steam the asparagus for 8–10 minutes, then put it in a large bowl. Meanwhile, gently fry the red pepper in 2 tbsp of the oil until soft, and add it to the asparagus with the eggs, herbs and remaining oil. Mix gently and season with black pepper.

globe artichoke

This classy vegetable has a special healing affinity with the liver, gallbladder and digestive system.

Since ancient times the globe artichoke has been used as a digestive aid and to ease liver and gallbladder disorders. Its main active constituent is cynarin, a phytochemical which enhances digestion, particularly following meals high in fat. Studies have shown that cynarin reduces nausea, abdominal pain, constipation and flatulence in people who regularly experience digestive problems. Artichokes may also help to lower high cholesterol levels by inhibiting the production of more cholesterol.

NUTRIENTS

Vitamins B1, B2, B3, B5, B6, C, E, K, beta-carotene; calcium, copper, iron, magnesium, manganese, phosphorus, potassium, selenium, zinc; fibre

SPICY ARTICHOKE DRESSING

**400g/14oz fresh globe
   artichokes or tinned
   artichoke hearts**
2 tbsp unrefined sunflower oil
1 tbsp lemon juice
½ clove garlic
1 tsp mild chilli powder
8 tbsp vegetable juice

If using fresh artichokes, break off the outer leaves and cut away the inner leaves. Scrape out and boil the hearts for about 20 minutes. If using tinned artichokes, put all the ingredients in a food processor and blend until creamy.

lettuce

NUTRIENTS

Vitamins B1, B3, B5, C, E, K, beta-carotene, biotin, folate; calcium, iodine, iron, magnesium, manganese, phosphorus, potassium, selenium, silica, zinc

A salad staple, lettuce helps to cleanse the blood, relax the nerves and eliminate excess fluid.

This leafy vegetable contains a natural sedative called lactucarium, which relaxes the nervous system and induces sleep. To treat insomnia, try drinking lettuce juice before going to bed. With its high potassium content, lettuce is also a mild diuretic, while its chlorophyll helps to detoxify the blood and liver. Other nutrients in lettuce include folic acid, important for preventing birth defects, and beta-carotene and vitamin C, two immunity-boosting vitamins, which help to keep colds at bay.

GREEN SALAD SUPREME

3 large handfuls of mixed lettuce leaves
½ cucumber, sliced
100g/3½oz feta cheese, cubed
1 avocado, peeled, pitted and chopped
2 tbsp salad cress
2 tbsp chopped chives
2 tbsp olive oil
1 tbsp cider vinegar
sea salt and ground black pepper to taste

Put all the ingredients in a large bowl, toss well and serve.

Choose darker coloured lettuce varieties over paler-looking ones, as they contain more nutrients.

radicchio

Also known as red chicory, this attractive, red-leaved vegetable adds antioxidant power to salads.

A mainstay in the Mediterranean diet, radicchio has long been praised for its blood-purifying effects. Moreover, it is among some of the highest-scoring vegetables for antioxidant activity. In particular, it is rich in anthocyanins, phytochemicals which help to strengthen blood capillaries and inhibit inflammation, making radicchio a beneficial food for circulatory problems and conditions such as asthma and arthritis. Additionally, radicchio contains intybin, a mild appetite stimulant, which aids digestion and liver function.

NUTRIENTS
Vitamins B1, B2, B3, B5, B6, C, E, K, beta-carotene, folate; calcium, copper, iron, magnesium, manganese, phosphorus, potassium, selenium, zinc

RADICCHIO WITH BEANS

1 radicchio
a handful of peanuts
1 tbsp chopped flat-leaf
  parsley
100g/3½oz fine green beans,
  trimmed and chopped
100g/3½oz broad beans
3 tbsp olive oil
juice of ½ lemon

Arrange the radicchio leaves in a large bowl with the peanuts and parsley. Steam the green beans for 8 minutes and the broad beans for 20 minutes, then add them to the salad. Mix the oil and lemon juice, pour it over the salad and toss well.

spinach

NUTRIENTS
Vitamins B3, B5, B6, C, E, K, beta-carotene, biotin, folate; calcium, chromium, iodine, iron, magnesium, manganese, phosphorus, potassium, selenium, sodium, zinc; fibre

This popular type of greens contains a powerhouse of nutrients that protect the body from numerous degenerative diseases.

Containing at least 13 different flavonoid antioxidants, spinach may reduce the risk of heart disease, stroke and several cancers. It is also rich in lutein, a carotenoid compound that helps to guard against age-related eye diseases. Furthermore, spinach is a superb food for the bones, as it provides calcium and magnesium as well as vitamin K, which is thought to play an important role in bone mineralization.

CHEESE AND SPINACH MELT

1 onion, chopped
1 tbsp olive oil
2 cloves garlic, crushed
55g/2oz/⅓ cup pine nuts
225g/8oz baby leaf spinach
250g/9oz cheese, grated

Gently fry the onion in the oil, add the garlic and pine nuts and stir in the spinach until it wilts. Drain off any excess liquid, then add the cheese, stirring until it melts. Use the mixture in pancakes, on toast or to stuff vegetables.

watercress

Packed with more than 15 vitamins and minerals, watercress has long enjoyed superfood status.

Weight for weight, watercress contains more calcium than milk, more iron than spinach and as much vitamin C as oranges, making it an excellent food for the bones, blood and immune system. It is also a fabulous source of lutein and zeaxanthin – types of carotenoids that reduce the risk of eye disease. Watercress also possesses a unique compound called PEITC, which has not only been found to inhibit the growth of cancer, but is thought to kill existing cancerous cells as well.

NUTRIENTS
Vitamins B1, B3, B5, B6, C, E, K, beta-carotene, biotin, folate; calcium, iodine, iron, magnesium, manganese, phosphorus, potassium, zinc

CARROT, ORANGE AND WATERCRESS SALAD

1 bunch watercress, trimmed
2 carrots, peeled and grated
1 orange, peeled and chopped
1 avocado, peeled, pitted and chopped
a handful of walnuts
1 tbsp chopped oregano
1 tbsp chopped parsley
2 tbsp unrefined sunflower oil
juice of ½ lemon
sea salt and ground black pepper

Put the watercress, carrots, orange, avocado, walnuts and herbs in a large bowl. Add the sunflower oil, lemon juice, salt and pepper and toss well. Serve immediately.

okra

NUTRIENTS
Vitamins B1, B3, B5, B6, C, K, beta-carotene, biotin, folate; calcium, iodine, iron, magnesium, manganese, phosphorus, potassium, selenium, zinc; fibre

Also known as lady's finger, okra is high in fibre, helping to regulate bowel function and encourage the growth of friendly bacteria in the gut.

Native to Africa, okra has found its way into many types of global cuisine including Indian, Caribbean and Middle Eastern cooking. Its main health attribute is its fibre content, which helps to stabilize blood sugar levels and lower high cholesterol, reducing the risk of heart disease. It also has a bulking effect in the large intestine, thereby preventing or alleviating constipation. Okra secretes a mucilaginous juice during cooking, which adds body when used to prepare curries, soups and sauces.

EASY OKRA

2 tbsp unrefined sunflower oil
1 onion, chopped
1 tsp crushed red chillies
1 tsp ground cumin
1 tsp turmeric
2 tbsp tomato purée
350g/12oz okra, trimmed and chopped

Heat the oil in a pan and gently fry the onion until soft. Add the chillies, cumin, turmeric and tomato purée, and stir for a minute or so. Add 300ml/ 10½fl oz/1¼ cups water and the okra, bring to the boil and simmer, covered, for about 12 minutes until tender. Serve as an accompaniment.

shiitake mushroom

This highly-prized mushroom has been revered in the Far East for thousands of years, both as a tasty food and a potent medicine.

Several therapeutic compounds have been identified in shiitake mushrooms. Lentinan not only stimulates the immune system, but appears to trigger the production of interferon, which has anti-viral and anti-cancer properties and is used in Japan to treat cancer, AIDS, diabetes, chronic fatigue syndrome and fibrocytic breast disease. Eritadenine, another component in shiitake, reduces cholesterol, while tyrosinase lowers blood pressure. Shiitake mushrooms are available either fresh or dried.

NUTRIENTS
Vitamins B1, B2, B3, B5, B6, C; calcium, copper, iron, magnesium, manganese, phosphorus, potassium, selenium, zinc; fibre; protein; omega-6 essential fatty acids

---

FRIED MUSHROOM SALAD

3 large handfuls of mixed salad leaves
1 bunch of watercress, trimmed
4 tbsp olive oil
450g/1lb shiitake mushrooms
8 cloves garlic, crushed
ground black pepper

Put the salad leaves and watercress in a bowl. Heat 3 tbsp of the oil in a pan and sauté the mushrooms and garlic until tender. Add the contents of the pan to the salad with the remaining oil. Toss well, season with black pepper and serve.

avocado

NUTRIENTS

Vitamins B1, B2, B3, B5, B6, C, E, K, beta-carotene, biotin, folate; calcium, copper, iodine, iron, magnesium, manganese, phosphorus, potassium, zinc; fibre; monounsaturated fats; lecithin

Contrary to popular belief, avocados can be helpful during a weight-loss programme.

Shunned by dieters because of their high calorie count, avocados may actually aid weight loss by satisfying hunger, improving metabolism and balancing blood sugar levels. Full of health-giving nutrients, they are an excellent source of vitamin E and healthy monounsaturated fats, which help to nourish the skin and protect against stroke and cardiovascular disease. Another type of fat in this delicious, creamy food is lecithin, which plays a role in improving brain function.

AVOCADO DIP

2 ripe avocados, peeled, pitted and chopped
½ onion, chopped
1 clove garlic, crushed
2 tbsp chopped fresh coriander
4 tomatoes, chopped
1 green chilli, deseeded and chopped
2 tbsp crème fraîche
1 tbsp fresh lime juice
pinch of black pepper

Put all the ingredients in a food processor and blend until creamy. To prevent the dip from going brown, place the avocado stone in it and cover with cling film.

Avocado can be used as a healthy spread in place of butter or margarine.

olive and olive oil

The regular consumption of olive oil in Mediterranean countries could explain the robust health enjoyed by many people who live there.

Rich in vitamin E and monounsaturated fats, olives and their oil have been found to lower high cholesterol, an effect thought to be linked to the phytosterols responsible for reducing cholesterol absorption from food. Olives also contain squalene, which has heart-protecting properties, oleoeuropein, which lowers high blood pressure and oleocanthal, which relieves inflammation. Olive oil can be used to soften wax inside the ears.

Choose "extra virgin" olive oil which contains the most antioxidants and nutrients.

NUTRIENTS
Vitamins E, K, beta-carotene; calcium, copper, iodine, iron, magnesium, manganese, phosphorus, potassium, selenium, zinc; monounsaturated fats

GREEK PASTA SALAD

300g/10½oz wholemeal pasta
3 tomatoes, chopped
½ cucumber, peeled and
  chopped
1 spring onion, trimmed and
  chopped
100g/3½oz black olives
55g/2oz feta cheese or dairy-
  free alternative, cubed
5 tbsp chopped parsley
3 tbsp olive oil
sea salt and ground black
  pepper to taste

Cook the pasta in boiling water until *al dente*, then drain. Transfer to a large bowl and add all the other ingredients. Mix well and serve.

cabbage

Often overlooked as a healing food, the humble cabbage has much to offer in therapeutic benefits.

NUTRIENTS
Vitamins B1, B3, B5, B6, C, E, K, U, beta-carotene, biotin, folate; calcium, iodine, iron, magnesium, manganese, phosphorus, potassium, selenium, zinc; fibre

STIR-FRIED CABBAGE WITH LEEKS

2 tbsp olive oil
½ Savoy cabbage, shredded
1 leek, trimmed and chopped
3 cloves garlic, crushed
ground black pepper

Heat the oil in a wok and stir-fry the cabbage, leek and garlic until cooked through. Season with black pepper and serve as a vegetable accompaniment.

FIGHTS CANCER

A member of the cruciferous food family, cabbage contains powerful anti-cancer compounds, namely indoles and sulforaphane. Recent studies have shown that people who eat at least three servings of cruciferous vegetables each week have a lower risk of prostate, colorectal and lung cancer. In addition, indoles help to deactivate oestrone, a dangerous form of oestrogen that is associated with breast cancer.

HEALS ULCERS

A substance unique to raw cabbage known as vitamin U or S-methylmethionine has had remarkable success in healing stomach and duodenal ulcers within as little as four days. Drinking just four glasses of raw cabbage juice every day appears to dramatically reduce the pain and healing time of gastro-intestinal ulcers. The amino acid glutamine, which has anti-inflammatory properties, may also contribute to this.

Cabbage leaves can be used for enhancing the healing process of leg ulcers, wounds and varicose veins when applied externally to the problem area. Mastitis or breast inflammation, often experienced by mothers when breast-feeding, may also be relieved in this way.

In addition, cabbage can be a useful aid for gastro-intestinal health – the German fermented cabbage product *sauerkraut* supports the digestive tract by promoting the growth of friendly bacteria in the gut.

SAVOY POTATO BAKE

1 tbsp olive oil
½ Savoy cabbage, shredded
3 large potatoes, peeled and
    diced
1 tbsp unhydrogenated
    margarine
sea salt and black pepper

Heat the oil and 2 tbsp water in a large pan and sauté the cabbage for 8 minutes. Meanwhile, steam the potatoes for 15 minutes, place in a bowl with the margarine, and mash. Add the cabbage, season with salt and pepper and mix well. Put the mixture in a dish and bake in a preheated oven at 200°C/400°F/Gas mark 6 for 40 minutes.

broccoli

NUTRIENTS
Vitamins B1, B3, B5, B6, C, E, K, beta-carotene, biotin, folate; calcium, iodine, iron, magnesium, manganese, phosphorus, potassium, zinc; fibre

Touted as a superfood, broccoli is crammed with an amazing blend of nutrients.

A relative of cabbage, broccoli contains potent anti-cancer compounds including diindolylmethane and sulforaphane, which work together to inhibit cancer growth. Diindolylmethane also promotes anti-viral and anti-bacterial activity, so eating broccoli regularly may help to protect against and fight off infections. Its other health benefits include calcium and magnesium, which promote bone-building; lutein and zeaxanthin, which reduce the risk of eye disease; and vitamin C which fortifies the immune system.

BROCCOLI POTAGE

1 tbsp olive oil
2 shallots, finely chopped
1 clove garlic, crushed
1 sweet potato, peeled and
  diced
1 tomato, chopped
750ml/26fl oz/3 cups vegetable
  stock
100g/3½oz broccoli, chopped
croutons

Heat the oil in a large pan and gently fry the shallots, garlic, sweet potato and tomato for a few minutes. Add the stock and broccoli, bring to the boil and simmer, covered, for 20 minutes. Pour the mixture into a blender and whiz until smooth. Tip back into the pan and heat through. Serve with croutons.

carrot

Known for its ability to aid night vision, this root vegetable can be used in both sweet and savoury dishes or pressed into a delicious, sweet juice.

Carrots are one of the richest sources of beta-carotene, a carotenoid which is converted into vitamin A in the body. This vitamin is required for normal vision, healthy-looking skin and effective reproductive function, as well as for helping the body to fight infections such as colds and bronchitis. Eating just two carrots a day appears to reduce high cholesterol levels. This is likely to be due to calcium pectate, a type of soluble fibre that provides them with their characteristic crunchiness.

NUTRIENTS

Vitamins B1, B3, B5, B6, C, E, K, beta-carotene, biotin, folate; calcium, iodine, iron, magnesium, manganese, phosphorus, potassium, selenium, zinc; fibre

CARROT AND CELERY COCKTAIL

10 large carrots, peeled
3 raw beetroot, peeled
2 celery sticks
2 green peppers, deseeded
200g/7oz spinach
a large handful of parsley

Cut the carrots, beetroot, celery and peppers into small chunks and press them through a juicer along with the spinach and parsley. Stir and drink immediately.

beetroot

NUTRIENTS

Vitamins B3, B5, C, folate,
beta-carotene; calcium, iodine,
iron, magnesium, manganese,
phosphorus, potassium, zinc; fibre;
carbohydrate

RAW BEETROOT SALAD

2 raw beetroot,
½ celeriac
1 carrot
2 tbsp sunflower seeds
1 tbsp chopped parsley
2 tbsp chopped chives
4 tbsp bio-yogurt
1 tbsp olive oil
1 tbsp lemon juice
sea salt and ground black
    pepper to taste

Peel and grate the beetroot,
celeriac and carrot and put
them in a large bowl with the
sunflower seeds and fresh
herbs. Mix together using your
hands. Then, add the remaining
ingredients and mix well.

Valued for its powerful detoxifying capabilities,
beetroot is a very effective internal cleanser.

Containing the powerful antioxidant betacyanin, which gives
this root vegetable its deep red colour, beetroot helps to cleanse
the liver, gallbladder and kidneys. Betacyanin also boosts the
activity of natural antioxidant enzymes in the body, which
protect cells against the dangers of free radical damage. A rich
source of natural sugars, beetroot provides easily digestible
carbohydrates for energy, while its dietary fibre content is
useful for preventing digestive problems.

To retain the
maximum amount of
nutrients and colour
in beetroot, peel
it after cooking.

Jerusalem artichoke

Sweet and nutty in flavour, Jerusalem artichokes are an excellent source of slow-releasing energy.

Not to be confused with the globe artichoke, the Jerusalem variety is an edible tuber whose brown knobbly appearance resembles ginger root. It's rich in inulin, a type of carbohydrate that does not elevate blood sugar levels, making it a helpful food for diabetics. Inulin also encourages the growth of friendly bacteria in the gut, thereby promoting the health of the digestive tract. Nutrient-wise, this vegetable contains good amounts of iron needed for the formation of red blood cells, while its potassium content provides a mild diuretic effect.

NUTRIENTS
Vitamins B1, B3, C, E, K, beta-carotene; copper, iron, magnesium, manganese, phosphorus, potassium, selenium; fibre; protein; complex carbohydrate

Although the Jerusalem artichoke is related to the sunflower, it grows well in cold climates.

ARTICHOKE CHIPS

1kg/2lb 4oz Jerusalem
   artichokes
juice of 2 lemons
3 tbsp olive oil
2 bay leaves
ground black pepper

Cut the artichokes into chips and put them in a roasting tray. Squeeze the lemon juice over, along with the olive oil. Add the bay leaves to the tray and cook in a preheated oven at 190°C/375°F/Gas mark 5 for about 40 minutes until soft and golden. Serve sprinkled with black pepper.

mooli

This mild-flavoured, giant white radish cleanses the liver and assists in the digestion of fats.

Mooli, or daikon as it's also called, is a long, white radish popular in Japanese, Chinese and Korean cuisines. Containing active enzymes, it is often served raw and grated as a side dish to aid the digestion of fatty or oily meals. Mooli also enhances liver detoxification and is said to help to break up catarrh. Being high in water and very low in calories, it's a perfect food for anyone on a weight-loss diet.

NUTRIENTS
Vitamin C; calcium, iron, magnesium, phosphorus, potassium; fibre

ORIENTAL COLESLAW

1 mooli, trimmed and peeled
3 carrots, peeled
½ white baby cabbage
2 spring onions, trimmed and chopped
1 tbsp gomasio (optional)
2 tbsp toasted sesame oil
1 tbsp rice vinegar
sea salt and ground black pepper

Grate the mooli, carrots and cabbage and put them in a large bowl. Add the remaining ingredients and mix well. Serve with noodles and a protein source such as fish or tofu.

024

eddo

High in complex carbohydrates and low in fat, eddoes make a tasty change to rice or potatoes.

Also known as taro root, eddoes are small, tropical root vegetables with a mild, nutty flavour. High in complex carbohydrates, they are an excellent energy food and offer a delicious alternative to potatoes but with a lower glycaemic index. They are also a good source of potassium, which gives them a mild diuretic action. Once peeled, eddoes can be boiled, steamed or roasted, or added to soups and casseroles.

NUTRIENTS

Vitamins B1, B3, B5, B6, C, E, K, beta-carotene, folate; calcium, copper, iron, magnesium, manganese, phosphorus, potassium, selenium, zinc; fibre; protein; complex carbohydrate

ROASTED CHILLI EDDOES

4 eddoes, peeled
3 tbsp olive oil
1 tsp chilli powder

Cut the eddoes into chunks and steam them for about 5 minutes. Transfer them to a roasting tray and sprinkle with the oil and chilli powder. Roast in a preheated oven at 220°C/425°F/Gas mark 7 for 30 minutes, turning them half-way through the cooking time.

025

potato

NUTRIENTS
Vitamins B1, B3, B5, B6, C, K, biotin, folate; calcium, iodine, iron, magnesium, manganese, phosphorus, potassium, selenium, zinc; fibre; protein; complex carbohydrate

The world's premier vegetable crop, potatoes are inexpensive, versatile and packed with health-giving nutrients.

Often shunned for their high carbohydrate content, potatoes are fattening only if fried or covered in butter. A good all-round source of nutrition, they contain B-vitamins needed for metabolism, potassium which helps to regulate the elimination of fluid and vitamin C, which boosts immunity. They also possess flavonoids, known for their anti-cancer and anti-inflammatory properties, as well as compounds called kukoamines, which lower blood pressure.

SCALLOPED POTATOES

4 potatoes, peeled and sliced
2 tbsp olive oil
sea salt and ground black pepper
200ml/7fl oz/¾ cup vegetable stock

Brush the potato slices with the oil, season and arrange in a casserole dish with the slices overlapping. Pour over the stock, cover with foil and cook in a preheated oven at 220°C/425°F/Gas mark 7 for 1 hour. Then remove the foil and cook for an extra 15 minutes or until the liquid has evaporated.

sweet potato

From soups, casseroles and salads to baby food and desserts, sweet potatoes add taste, valuable nutrients and colour to any meal.

Orange-fleshed sweet potatoes are probably best known for their rich concentration of beta-carotene, which is converted into vitamin A in the body. This nutrient plays an important role in vision, bone growth, reproduction and keeping the lining of the digestive and respiratory tracts healthy. Sweet potatoes are also low in fat and loaded with potassium, which helps to maintain fluid balance in cells. Despite the name "sweet", this vegetable contains blood-sugar-regulating properties and is considered to be a useful food for diabetics.

NUTRIENTS
Vitamins B1, B3, B5, C, E, beta-carotene, biotin, folate; calcium, iodine, iron, magnesium, manganese, phosphorus, potassium, selenium, zinc; fibre; protein; complex carbohydrate

SWEET POTATO MASH

4 sweet potatoes, peeled and chopped
3 carrots, peeled and chopped
150g/5½oz frozen garden peas
2 tbsp butter or unhydrogenated margarine
sea salt and ground black pepper

Steam the sweet potatoes, carrots and peas for 20–25 minutes until soft. Transfer to a bowl, add the butter or margarine and salt and pepper, and mash until creamy. Serve instead of mashed regular potatoes.

yam

NUTRIENTS
Vitamins B1, B3, B5, B6, C, E, biotin, folate; calcium, iodine, iron, magnesium, manganese, phosphorus, potassium, selenium, zinc; fibre; complex carbohydrate

An excellent power food, yam is a delicious and sustaining form of slow-releasing carbohydrate.

Used in a similar way to potatoes, yams have a lower glycaemic index and so provide a more sustained form of energy. This makes them a good source of carbohydrate for diabetics and weight-watchers. Yams are high in potassium and low in sodium, which helps to regulate fluid balance. Their vitamin C and B6 content and dietary fibre all contribute to good health.

YAM HOT POT

2 tbsp olive oil
1 onion, chopped
1 clove garlic, crushed
½ yam, peeled and chopped
2 carrots, peeled and chopped
1 courgette, chopped
2 celery sticks, chopped
1 tsp paprika
300ml/10½fl oz/1¼ cups
vegetable stock
1 tbsp chopped parsley

Heat the oil in a pan and gently fry the onion. Add the garlic, vegetables and paprika, and stir for 2 minutes. Add the stock, bring to the boil and simmer, covered, for 15 minutes. Add the parsley just before serving.

horseradish

Used as a medicine in the Middle Ages, horseradish has anti-bacterial, diuretic and stimulant properties.

The kick and aroma of horseradish are almost unnoticeable until it is cut or grated and its volatile oils are released. These oils, particularly mustard oil, have natural antibiotic properties that can help to treat various ailments, including respiratory tract infections such as coughs and sinus congestion, and urinary tract infections. This root vegetable stimulates the digestion and is an effective diuretic. It also promotes perspiration, making it useful for cold and flu relief.

NUTRIENTS
Vitamins B3, C, K, beta-carotene, folate; calcium, iron, magnesium, phosphorus, potassium, selenium, zinc

TOFU AND HORSERADISH SAUCE

250g/9oz tofu
2 heaped tbsp grated
    horseradish
1 tsp white miso
3 tbsp unrefined sunflower oil
sea salt to taste

Put all the ingredients with 250ml/9fl oz/1 cup water in a food processor and blend until smooth and creamy. This sauce is particularly delicious served with fish or vegetables.

Mix grated horseradish with vinegar to prevent it from browning and becoming bitter.

butternut squash

NUTRIENTS
Vitamins B1, B3, B5, B6, C, E, K,
beta-carotene, folate; calcium,
copper, iron, magnesium,
phosphorus, potassium, selenium,
zinc; fibre; protein; complex
carbohydrate

A popular variety of winter squash, this vegetable is a great source of energy-sustaining carbohydrates.

Butternut squash is particularly high in beta-carotene, which is converted into vitamin A in the body and needed for healthy skin and normal immune, digestive and respiratory tract function. It also contains other carotenoids, including beta-cryptoxanthin, which may significantly lower the risk of lung cancer. Extracts from squash have also been found to reduce the symptoms of benign prostatic hyperplasia, a condition of the prostate gland.

ROASTED BUTTERNUT SQUASH

1 butternut squash
1 tbsp olive oil
sea salt and ground black
pepper

Cut the squash in half lengthways, remove the seeds and brush the flesh with the oil. Cook face-down in a preheated oven at 220°C/425°F/Gas mark 7 for 45 minutes until soft. Once cooked, season to taste with the salt and pepper.

030

agar-agar

This bland, calorie-free seaweed offers a fabulous vegetarian alternative to gelatine for the making of jellies and aspics.

Rich in trace minerals, agar-agar is traditionally used in Japan to help soothe the digestive tract and to relieve constipation. Its high fibre content helps to lower raised cholesterol and suppresses the appetite, making it an ideal food for anyone wanting to lose weight. The main culinary function of this seaweed is as a gelling agent, setting liquids at room temperature. However, it will not set in vinegar or in any foods containing oxalic acid, such as chocolate, rhubarb and spinach.

NUTRIENTS
Vitamins B2, B3, B5, B6, E, K, folate; calcium, copper, iodine, iron, magnesium, manganese, phosphorus, potassium, selenium, zinc; fibre

REAL FRUIT JELLY

400g/14oz soft fruit, chopped (such as peaches, strawberries, grapes)
600ml/21fl oz/2⅓ cups white grape juice
4 tbsp agar-agar flakes

Place the chopped fruit in a large heatproof glass bowl and set aside. Put the grape juice and agar-agar in a pan, bring to the boil and simmer for a few minutes while stirring, until the agar-agar has dissolved. Pour the liquid over the chopped fruit and leave to cool. Once set, store in the fridge.

kombu

NUTRIENTS
Vitamins B1, B2, B3, B12, C,
beta-carotene; calcium, iodine,
iron, magnesium, phosphorus,
potassium, sodium; fibre; protein

In Japan, this highly nutritious sea vegetable is often used to add flavour to soups, broths and stocks.

Laden with protein and minerals such as calcium, magnesium, potassium, iodine and iron, kombu improves the nutritional value of any meal into which it is incorporated. It also acts as a tenderizer and is often added to beans to reduce their cooking time and make them easier to digest.

DESTROYS CONTAMINANTS
Heavy metals are common contaminants that can get absorbed into the body where they are stored in organs and tissues. Kombu possesses a fibre molecule called alginic acid which is able to bind to heavy metals such as cadmium, mercury and lead and carry them out of the system.

FIGHTS MANY ILLNESSES
A recently discovered substance in kombu called fucoidan has been found to make cancer cells self-destruct. This compound has now been extracted from the seaweed and is available as a nutritional supplement.

Due to kombu's excellent nutrient profile and cleansing abilities, it's claimed to offer relief in a range of health conditions

---

KOMBU TOMATO STOCK

1 strip dried kombu
6 sun-dried tomatoes

Soak the kombu and tomatoes in 1 litre/35fl oz/4 cups water for 30 minutes, then bring to the boil and simmer for 5 minutes. Remove the kombu and tomatoes. Use the liquid for any recipe that calls for stock. The kombu can be reused to make more stock or added to beans or casseroles during cooking to enhance the flavour.

from rheumatism, arthritis and high blood pressure to goitre caused by an under-active thyroid.

Being a rich source of glutamic acid – a natural form of the synthetic flavour-enhancer monosodium glutamate (MSG) – kombu is extremely useful when added to stocks, soups, stews and broths, where it enhances and brings out the flavours of other ingredients.

CANNELLINI KOMBU BEAN POT

200g/7oz cannellini beans
1 strip dried kombu
½ leek, trimmed and chopped
½ red pepper, deseeded and chopped
200g/7oz spinach, chopped

Soak the beans overnight in plenty of cold water. Next day, drain, place in a pan and cover with 1 litre/35fl oz/4 cups water. Add the kombu, then bring to the boil and simmer, covered, for about 2 hours until the beans are soft. Add the leek, red pepper and spinach and cook for a further 15 minutes. Mix well and serve.

nori

Vitamins B1, B3, B5, B6, C, E, K, beta-carotene, folate; calcium, copper, iron, magnesium, phosphorus, potassium, selenium, zinc; fibre; protein; complex carbohydrate

Just one dried sheet of nori seaweed provides the body with as much vitamin A as three eggs.

Used in sushi-making, this "fishy"-tasting seaweed has been cultivated in Japan for over a thousand years. An excellent source of protein, nori helps with growth and tissue repair, and its calcium and iron content nourishes the bones and blood. Particularly high in beta-carotene, nori may help to promote skin health, boost the immune system and slow down eye disease. It also contains vitamin B12, which is rarely found in the plant world, making it an ideal food for strict vegetarians.

NORI POTATO FRITTERS

2 large potatoes, peeled and coarsely grated
1 onion, finely chopped
4 free-range eggs
5 tbsp nori flakes
1 tbsp ground mustard seeds
olive oil for shallow frying

Using your hands, squeeze as much of the juice from the grated potatoes as possible, then put them in a bowl and mix them with the onion, eggs, nori and mustard seed. Warm the oil in a frying pan, adding the mixture when the oil is hot. Flatten each fritter with a fork and for a few minutes cook on both sides until golden.

wakame

A green leafy sea vegetable, wakame can be soaked and used in salads in place of lettuce.

Traditionally added to miso soup, wakame is mild in flavour and is one of the most popular sea vegetables. It's an excellent source of potassium and may improve heart health by keeping high blood pressure in check. It's also an outstanding source of calcium needed for bone maintenance, and magnesium for relieving stress and muscle tension. In Japan, wakame is used as a blood purifier and is also valued for its nourishing effect on the hair and skin.

NUTRIENTS
Vitamins B3, B5, C, E, K, beta-carotene, folate; calcium, iodine, iron, magnesium, manganese, phosphorus, potassium, selenium, sodium; fibre; protein; omega-3 essential fatty acids

---

WAKAME NOODLE BROTH

2 tbsp sesame oil
1 clove garlic, crushed
2 celery sticks, chopped
1 litre/35fl oz/4 cups vegetable stock
1 tbsp miso
2 carrots, peeled and diced
8 strips wakame, chopped
50g/1¾oz dried noodles

Put all the ingredients (except the noodles) in a large pan, and bring to the boil, stirring until the miso has dissolved. Simmer, covered, for 30 minutes. Add the noodles and cook for a further few minutes until they are cooked through. Serve immediately.

dulse

NUTRIENTS

Vitamins B1, B2, B3, B6, C, beta-carotene; calcium, iodine, iron, magnesium, phosphorus, potassium, sodium, zinc; fibre; protein

This purple-red, peppery seaweed can be added to salads, soups and casseroles or dry-roasted over an open flame and used as a garnish.

Full of potassium which helps to relieve fluid retention, dulse is also the most iron-rich of the edible seaweeds, making it an excellent food for combating anaemia. Like most sea vegetables, it's high in iodine, which is needed to make the thyroid hormone and to help to regulate the thyroid gland. A lack of iodine in the diet can result in an under-active thyroid, causing fatigue and weight gain. Eaten in small amounts, dulse is thought to be an effective remedy for sea sickness.

SEA SALAD

3 tbsp dulse, rinsed
2 handfuls of mixed salad leaves
½ cucumber, peeled and chopped
1 spring onion, trimmed and chopped
2 tbsp sesame oil
1 tbsp rice vinegar
1 tbsp sesame seeds

Soak the dulse in water for about 3 minutes, then drain and cut it into pieces with scissors. Put it in a large bowl along with the salad leaves, cucumber and spring onion. Add the sesame oil and rice vinegar, toss well and serve sprinkled with sesame seeds.

hijiki

This black, wiry sea vegetable has a rich flavour and is delicious when added to rice, beans or stir-fries.

Rich in a broad spectrum of minerals, hijiki is thought to play a contributory role to the thick, shiny hair enjoyed by many Japanese people. It's a superb bone-builder, containing more calcium than any other sea vegetable, and if included in the diet several times a week, it may help to prevent osteoporosis and other bone diseases. Hijiki is also high in fibre, which helps to regulate blood sugar levels and lower elevated cholesterol. Like kombu, it contains the cancer-busting compound, fucoidan.

NUTRIENTS

Vitamins B1, B2, B3, B12, beta-carotene; calcium, iodine, iron, phosphorus, potassium, sodium; fibre; protein

SCRAMBLED EGGS WITH HIJIKI

2 heaped tbsp hijiki
1 tbsp olive oil
4 free-range eggs
6 cherry tomatoes, sliced
2 tbsp finely chopped chives
1 tsp ground mustard seeds
1 clove garlic, crushed
sea salt and ground black
   pepper to taste

Soak the hijiki in water for 15 minutes, then drain and sauté in the oil for about 8 minutes. Meanwhile, beat the eggs in a bowl and add the remaining ingredients. Pour the mixture over the hijiki and cook, stirring frequently until the eggs have thickened but are still soft.

© ✋ ◎ ◒ ◓ ◐ ♡ ◒ ◑ 🌀 ❀

apple

NUTRIENTS

Vitamins B3, C, E, K, beta-carotene, biotin, folate; calcium, chromium, iron, magnesium, manganese, phosphorus, potassium, zinc; fibre; carbohydrate

With more varieties now available than ever before, apples are a delicious source of health benefits.

The old adage "an apple a day keeps the doctor away" could well hold true. According to studies, apples may reduce the risk of several common cancers, as well as protect the brain from the damage that causes conditions such as Alzheimer's and Parkinson's disease. Antioxidant compounds in the skin of apples, in particular quercetin, epicatechin and procyanidin, are thought to be responsible for this protective action. Apples also contain a soluble fibre called pectin, which lowers high cholesterol levels and regulates digestive function.

APPLE AND APRICOT CRUMBLE

200ml/7fl oz/¾ cup apple juice
6 apples, peeled, cored and
    chopped
284g/9¾oz sugar-free apricot
    jam
55g/2oz unhydrogenated
    margarine
115g/4oz/1 cup rolled oats
3 tbsp oatbran

Put the apple juice in a pan and bring to the boil. Add the apples and simmer, covered, until the liquid evaporates. Mash, add the jam, and spread in an oven-proof dish. Work the margarine into the oats and oatbran to form a crumble. Spoon it over the fruit and bake at 180°C/350°F/Gas mark 4 for about 30 minutes.

pear

Besides making an ideal dessert or snack, pears and pear juice can be used to sweeten cakes and cereals instead of sugar.

Pears are often given as a baby's first fruit, as they are the least likely to cause an allergic reaction. This also makes them one of the best fruits for people with multiple food allergies. The insoluble fibre in pears helps to eliminate cholesterol from the body, which is useful for those at risk of heart disease. Pears also regulate digestion and their vitamin C and folate content boost immunity.

NUTRIENTS

Vitamins B3, C, E, K, beta-carotene, biotin, folate; calcium, iodine, iron, magnesium, phosphorus, potassium, zinc; fibre; carbohydrate

PEARS IN CAROB SAUCE

300ml/10½fl oz/1¼ cups white grape juice
6 pears, peeled, cored and cut in half lengthways
280g/10oz tofu
3 tbsp brown rice syrup
2 tbsp hazelnut butter
1 tsp carob powder
1 tsp grain coffee substitute
2 tbsp unrefined sunflower oil

Put two-thirds of the grape juice in a pan and bring to the boil. Add the pears and simmer, covered, for 8 minutes until the liquid has evaporated. Divide into four dessert bowls. Put the remaining juice and ingredients in a food processor and blend until creamy. Serve with the cooked pears.

banana

Creamy, sweet and satisfying, bananas are a much-loved fruit for everyone from toddlers to seniors.

Concentrated in easily-digestible carbohydrates and low in fat, bananas are valued for their instant and sustained energy boost. One of the best sources of potassium, they offer protection against high blood pressure and fluid retention and are particularly useful after a bout of diarrhoea, which can cause potassium loss. Bananas are also high in tryptophan, an amino acid that the body converts into serotonin, a brain chemical known to improve mood and encourage relaxation.

Do not refrigerate unripe bananas as they will never ripen.

BANANA MILKSHAKE

2 bananas, chopped
500ml/17fl oz/2 cups soya milk
or milk of your choice
1 tbsp maple syrup
1 tbsp natural vanilla extract
1 tsp ground nutmeg

Put the first four ingredients in a blender and blend until smooth. Serve chilled, sprinkled with the nutmeg.

grape

Grapes are very effective at eliminating toxins from the body and cleansing the blood and intestines.

In folk medicine, grapes were used to purify the blood, clean the digestive system and counter liver and kidney disorders. Their high water and fibre content certainly makes them a useful detoxifying agent. Grapes also contain antioxidants that fight cancer and promote cardiovascular function, including resveratrol found specifically in red grapes. This compound, together with pterostilbene and saponins, aids heart health by reducing the risk of blood clots and relaxing blood vessels.

NUTRIENTS

Vitamins B3, B6, C, K, beta-carotene, biotin, folate; calcium, copper, iodine, iron, magnesium, manganese, phosphorus, potassium, selenium, zinc; fibre; carbohydrate

NON-ALCOHOLIC RED GRAPE SANGRIA

1 apple
3 oranges
1 lime
1 lemon
1 tbsp agave syrup
1litre/35fl oz/4 cups red grape juice

Slice the apple and one orange and put them in a glass pitcher. Juice the remaining fruit and add to the pitcher along with the agave syrup and grape juice. Serve chilled with ice.

cherry

040

NUTRIENTS
Vitamins B3, B5, C, beta-carotene, biotin, folate; calcium, iron, magnesium, manganese, phosphorus, potassium, selenium; fibre; carbohydrate

---

CHERRY PARFAIT

300g/10½oz cherries, pitted
500g/1lb 2oz/2 cups bio-yogurt
  or soya yogurt
150g/5½oz crunchy granola
  cereal
2 tbsp desiccated coconut,
  plus extra to serve
1 tbsp sugar-free cherry jam
  (optional)

Put all the ingredients in a food processor and blend until creamy. Serve chilled, sprinkled with extra coconut.

Besides helping to ease pain and inflammation, the naturally-occurring melatonin found in this delicious summer fruit may help to restore irregular sleep patterns.

Packed with anthocyanins, antioxidants which give this fruit its red hue, cherries help to shut down certain enzymes that cause inflammation, so can prevent many kinds of pain. In particular they seem to offer relief from gout – a form of arthritis that occurs when uric acid crystals accumulate in joints, leading to pain and inflammation. In studies, cherries have been found to significantly decrease uric acid levels, so limiting the formation of the gout-inducing crystals.

Cherries can also help to ease pain caused by both osteoarthritis and rheumatoid arthritis, as well as fibromyalgia – pain in the fibrous tissues of the body such as the muscles, tendons and ligaments.

SLEEP ENHANCERS
Other antioxidants in cherries include superoxide dismutase (useful in joint, respiratory and gastrointestinal health) and melatonin – one of the most potent known free radical scavengers ever discovered. Low melatonin levels have been

associated with sleep disturbances such as insomnia, so cherries could be a useful source of this compound, possibly aiding sleep. Melatonin is also important for the function of the immune system.

Proanthocyanidins, another antioxidant found in cherries, have anti-inflammatory activity and can strengthen blood vessels and slow down the ageing process of the skin.

CHERRY AND RHUBARB COMPOTE

400g/14oz cherries, pitted
3 rhubarb sticks, chopped
3 tbsp apple juice
2 tbsp fruit sugar
yogurt

Put all the ingredients, except the yogurt, in a pan. Bring to the boil and simmer, covered, for about 8 minutes, stirring occasionally. Serve with bio-yogurt.

date

NUTRIENTS

Vitamins B3, B5, B6, C, K, beta-carotene, biotin, folate; calcium, copper, iodine, iron, magnesium, manganese, phosphorus, potassium, selenium, zinc; fibre; carbohydrate

Available fresh or dried, dates are full of natural sweetness, and make a much healthier snack than refined carbohydrate treats.

Naturally sweet and chewy, dates are perfect for satisfying a sweet tooth without resorting to sugar. They are an excellent source of potassium, important for maintaining fluid and electrolyte balance in the body, and are loaded with fibre, which helps regulate bowel function. The tannin content of dates provides them with an astringent effect, which is of particular benefit for intestinal problems such as diarrhoea. As a traditional remedy it is believed that dates can counteract alcohol intoxication.

STUFFED DATES

175g/6oz/1¾ cups ground almonds
4 tbsp brown rice syrup
1 tbsp natural almond extract
12 fresh pitted dates
12 almonds (or nuts of your choice)

Combine the ground almonds, brown rice syrup and almond extract together until a paste is formed. Cut the dates almost in half lengthways, being careful not to cut all the way through, and stuff each one with almond paste. Top each date with an almond to serve.

fig

Front-runners in the calcium stakes, figs can help to boost levels of this key bone-building mineral.

Although it's not apparent, figs are one of the best sources of calcium, vital for bone growth in children and bone density in adults. They also contain more fibre than any other dried or fresh fruit, aiding satiety by promoting a feeling of fullness in the stomach and helping to balance blood sugar levels. In addition, their high fibre content provides a laxative effect, which is of benefit to those who suffer from chronic constipation.

NUTRIENTS

Vitamins B3, B5, B6, C, beta-carotene, biotin, folate; calcium, copper, iodine, iron, magnesium, manganese, phosphorus, potassium, zinc; fibre; carbohydrate

HONEY-BAKED FIGS

8 fresh figs
4 tbsp clear honey
4 tbsp chopped nuts
8 tbsp Greek bio-yogurt

Trim the end of the stalks off the figs, then cut a cross in the top of each one to open them up. Mix together the honey and nuts, and spoon the mixture into the top of the figs. Place them in an oven-proof dish and cook in a preheated oven at 190°C/375°F/Gas mark 5 for about 15 minutes until the figs are soft. Serve with the yogurt.

prune

NUTRIENTS
Vitamins B2, B3, B5, B6,
beta-carotene, folate; calcium,
copper, iodine, iron, magnesium,
manganese, phosphorus,
potassium, selenium, zinc; fibre;
carbohydrate

With one of the highest antioxidant rankings of all fruit, there's much more to prunes than their ability to prevent constipation.

Prunes are dried plums, both of which have made headlines in relation to their rich phytochemical content, namely neochlorogenic and chlorogenic acids. These antioxidant compounds help to neutralize hazardous free radicals in the body, protecting cells from damage and slowing down the ageing process. Eating prunes is also a sweet way of increasing beta-carotene, potassium, iron and fibre intake. In addition, prunes contain a natural laxative called diphenylisatin, which is why they are so useful for keeping the bowel regular.

AROMATIC STEWED PRUNES

250g/9oz soft pitted prunes
juice of 2 oranges
pinch of ground cinnamon

Put the prunes in a pan with the orange juice and cinnamon, bring to the boil then simmer, covered, for about 15 minutes. Serve with yogurt for breakfast or as a dessert.

044

blueberry

Blueberries are the number one fruit for helping to protect cells from free radical damage and ageing.

According to research, blueberries rank top in antioxidant activity compared to 40 other fresh fruit and vegetables. They get their beautiful blue colour from anthocyanins, potent antioxidants that help to neutralize cancer-forming substances in the body. Their other phytochemicals include proanthocyanidins, which protect the eyes, skin and blood vessels, and pterostilbene, which has anti-diabetic and cholesterol-lowering properties and may reduce cognitive decline. Blueberries are a fine source of vitamin C and they also contain anti-bacterial agents.

NUTRIENTS
Vitamins B3, B5, C, K, beta-carotene, folate; calcium, iron, magnesium, manganese, phosphorus, potassium, selenium, zinc; fibre; carbohydrate

---

BLUEBERRY FOOL

500g/1lb 2oz tofu
200ml/7fl oz/¾ cup apple juice
250g/9oz blueberries plus
    extra to serve
300ml/10½fl oz/1¼ cups
    agave syrup
100ml/3½fl oz/⅓ cup unrefined
    sunflower oil
1 tsp natural vanilla extract

Put the tofu and apple juice in a food processor and blend until smooth. Add the remaining ingredients and continue to blend until thick and creamy. Spoon into dessert glasses and serve chilled, decorated with a few blueberries on the top.

cranberry

NUTRIENTS

Vitamins B5, C, K, beta-carotene, folate; calcium, iron, magnesium, phosphorus, potassium, selenium; fibre; carbohydrate

---

CRANBERRY AND BANANA SMOOTHIE

300ml/10½fl oz/1¼ cups unsweetened cranberry juice
300ml/10½fl oz/1¼ cups white grape juice
2 bananas, chopped
10 strawberries, hulled
400g/14oz/1⅔ cups bio-yogurt or soya yogurt
3 tbsp honey

Put all the ingredients in a blender and whiz until smooth. Drink immediately.

Research has now confirmed the commonly believed folk wisdom that cranberries can prevent and treat urinary tract infections.

A popular remedy for treating cystitis, cranberries contain components that interfere with the adherence of bacteria to the lining of the urinary tract, allowing them to be flushed out more easily. Other compounds in this berry have been found to inhibit plaque-causing bacteria in the mouth, which causes tooth decay and gum disease. Cranberries also promote powerful anti-cancer activity and can combat kidney stone formation.

Look for cranberry juices that are sweetened with apple juice rather than sugar.

raspberry

Delicious and extremely nutritious, raspberries make a handy, health-giving alternative to sweets.

Bursting with antioxidants, the regular consumption of raspberries protects against many conditions, including inflammatory diseases, allergies, cardiovascular disease, age-related cognitive decline and cancer. They are particularly high in ellagic acid, which is thought to lower high cholesterol, reduce the risk of heart disease and promote the healing of wounds. On top of this, raspberries possess anti-bacterial properties, are an excellent source of vitamin C and are a rich source of fibre.

NUTRIENTS

Vitamins B3, B5, C, E, K, beta-carotene, biotin, folate; calcium, copper, iodine, iron, magnesium, manganese, phosphorus, potassium, selenium, zinc; fibre; carbohydrate

RASPBERRY COULIS

450g/1lb raspberries
1 tbsp fruit sugar
1 tsp lemon juice

Put all the ingredients in a food processor and blend. Pour the mixture through a fine sieve into a bowl, pressing on the solids. Serve the sauce on top of ice-cream or other desserts.

goji berry

In China, it is said that eating a handful of goji berries each morning will lift your mood and make you feel happy for the entire day.

Only available in their dried state outside of their production regions of China, Tibet and Mongolia, these vibrant orange-red berries are claimed to be one of the world's most powerful anti-ageing foods. Besides containing a remarkable range of essential nutrients, they possess several phytochemicals, including zeaxanthin, which protects against eye disease, solavetivone, an anti-bacterial agent, and physalin, an anti-leukaemia compound. The berries also supply special polysaccharides, which have antioxidant properties and can enhance immunity.

NUTRIENTS

Vitamins B1, B2, B6, C, E, beta-carotene, folate; calcium, iron, phosphorus, potassium, selenium, zinc; fibre; protein; carbohydrate; omega-3 and omega-6 essential fatty acids

LUXURY TRAIL MIX

Mix together 2 handfuls of goji berries with a handful of each of the following: sunflower seeds, pumpkin seeds, almonds, pine nuts, raisins, chopped dried dates, chopped dried banana and coconut shreds – plus any other favourite dried fruit or nuts. This makes a tasty, power-packed snack.

açai berry

With their spectacular nutritional and antioxidant profile, these berries may be one of the healthiest foods on the planet.

Native to the Amazon rainforest, açai berries (pronounced "a-sigh-ee") deteriorate quickly after harvesting, so are normally available only as a juice or fruit pulp to non-locals. They have recently created a stir because of their incredible nutritional content, which includes protein, monounsaturated fats, omega-6 and omega-3 essential fatty acids and many vitamins and minerals. Even more impressive is the fruit's phytochemical content: beta-sitosterol which reduces cholesterol; numerous antioxidants, such as anthocyanins which have anti-cancer and anti-inflammatory properties; and proanthocyanidins, which strengthen blood vessels.

NUTRIENTS
Vitamins B1, B2, B3, C, E, beta-carotene; calcium, copper, magnesium, phosphorus, potassium, zinc; fibre; protein; carbohydrate; monounsaturated fats, omega-3 and omega-6 essential fatty acids

---

AÇAI-BLUEBERRY WHIZ

300ml/10½fl oz/1¼ cups açai juice
600ml/21fl oz/2⅓ cups apple juice
200g/7oz blueberries
6 strawberries, hulled

Put all the ingredients in a blender and whiz until smooth. Drink immediately.

tangerine

NUTRIENTS

Vitamins B3, B5, C, E, K, beta-carotene, biotin, folate; calcium, iodine, iron, magnesium, phosphorus, potassium, selenium, zinc; fibre; carbohydrate

EXOTIC FRUIT MEDLEY

2 tangerines, peeled and segmented
2 mangoes, peeled, pitted and chopped
2 kiwi fruit, peeled and chopped
1 papaya, peeled and chopped
¼ pineapple, peeled and chopped
a handful of blueberries
juice of 1 lime
1 tbsp agave syrup

Put all the fruit in a large bowl. Add the lime juice and agave syrup and mix. Serve with yogurt, crème fraîche or a dairy-free alternative.

Ward off winter colds and flu with this juicy citrus fruit, which is high in immunity-boosting vitamin C.

This sweet and tangy citrus fruit is a cross between a mandarin and a bitter orange. It's an excellent source of both vitamin C and beta-carotene, important nutrients for skin maintenance and immune function, and also contains folic acid, which is needed to make red blood cells. Additionally, tangerines are endowed with three phytochemicals: hesperidin, a flavonoid that protects the heart, and tangeritin and limonene, which have been found to guard against various forms of cancer.

grapefruit

This sharp-tasting citrus fruit may help healthy weight reduction by boosting the metabolism.

Grapefruits come in shades from white to red. The pink and red ones are coloured by lycopene, a carotenoid with anti-cancer properties. Consumed first thing in the morning, grapefruit can prevent constipation, while eaten before a meal it stimulates the taste buds. Its low calorie count and glycaemic index make it useful for weight loss, along with its metabolism-stimulating action, which helps to burn fat. Grapefruit also contains vitamin C, as well as pectin to lower cholesterol, and bioflavonoids to strengthen blood capillaries.

NUTRIENTS

Vitamins B3, B5, C, E, beta-carotene, biotin, folate; calcium, iodine, iron, magnesium, phosphorus, potassium; fibre; carbohydrate

CITRUS FRUIT SALAD

3 large handfuls of mixed salad leaves
2 tbsp chopped parsley
1 tbsp chopped coriander
1 tbsp sunflower seeds
½ pink grapefruit
1 tbsp olive oil
1 tbsp lemon juice
1 tbsp orange juice

Put the salad leaves, parsley, coriander and sunflower seeds in a large bowl. Cut the grapefruit into segments and add them to the bowl. Drizzle the olive oil and citrus juices over the salad, then gently toss and serve immediately.

lemon

NUTRIENTS
Vitamins B3, B5, B6, C, E, beta-carotene, biotin, folate; calcium, copper, iodine, iron, magnesium, manganese, phosphorus, potassium, selenium, zinc; fibre; carbohydrate

Hot water with lemon juice and honey is one of the best natural remedies for soothing a sore throat.

Although lemons are not snack material, their health benefits can be reaped by using their freshly squeezed juice in salad dressings or as a flavouring agent in drinks and baked goods. Their high vitamin C content, along with natural antiseptic properties, makes them an effective remedy for sore throats, colds, flu and other infections. Lemons also stimulate the gall bladder, which in turn aids liver and digestive function. A compound called limonene, which also has anti-cancer activity is responsible for this effect.

SUGAR-FREE LEMONADE

750ml/26fl oz/3 cups carbonated water
600ml/21fl oz/2⅓ cups white grape juice
juice of 3 lemons
1 tbsp agave syrup

Put all the ingredients in a glass pitcher and stir. Serve chilled with plenty of ice.

052

guava

With their rich aroma and vibrant creamy flesh, guavas are delectable in home-made smoothies.

NUTRIENTS

Vitamins B3, B5, B6, C, E, beta-carotene, biotin, folate; calcium, copper, iodine, iron, magnesium, manganese, phosphorus, potassium, selenium, zinc; fibre; carbohydrate

The flavour of this small tropical fruit has been described as a cross between strawberry, pear and pineapple. Containing more vitamin C than citrus fruit, guavas help bolster the immune system, while their excellent beta-carotene content promotes healthy eyes and skin. They are also a good source of calcium, which is needed by the skeletal system, and are traditionally used to treat diarrhoea. According to studies, guavas have blood sugar-lowering properties that may be of benefit to people with diabetes.

MANGO-GUAVA LASSI

1 mango, peeled, pitted and chopped
1 guava, chopped
400ml/14fl oz/ 1½ cups apple juice
200ml/7fl oz/¾ cup milk or soya milk
200ml/7fl oz/¾ cup rice milk
1 tsp ground cardamom, plus extra for sprinkling

Put all the ingredients in a blender and blend until smooth. Sprinkle with a pinch of ground cardamom and drink immediately.

pomegranate

NUTRIENTS
Vitamins B3, B5, B6, C, E, beta-carotene, biotin, folate; calcium, copper, iron, magnesium, phosphorus, potassium, selenium, zinc; fibre; carbohydrate

Steeped in symbolism since ancient times, pomegranate now has superfood status, thanks to recent research into its healing attributes.

The edible seed clusters can make eating this fruit tricky, although with so many health rewards on offer, it's well worth the effort. Pomegranate is abundant in antioxidants called punicalagins, which have been shown to prevent several forms of cancer by protecting the body against free radicals, which can damage

> To remove seeds from a pomegranate, tap it on the skin side with a wooden spoon until they fall out.

FRUIT SALAD WITH POMEGRANATE

1 pomegranate
medium bunch white seedless grapes, destalked
150g/5½oz strawberries, hulled and chopped
1 banana, chopped
1 peach, pitted and chopped
100g/3½oz blueberries
4 tbsp fruit juice of choice
1 tbsp lemon juice
1 tbsp clear honey
pinch of ground nutmeg

Scoop out the seeds from the pomegranate and put them in a bowl along with the other fruit. Combine the fruit juice, lemon juice and honey, pour it over the fruit and mix gently. Serve sprinkled with the nutmeg.

cells. In fact, according to studies, one glass of pomegranate juice contains almost three times as many antioxidants as the same amount of red wine, green tea or orange juice.

A HEALTHY HEART

In relation to heart disease, pomegranate not only lowers high blood pressure but helps to fight LDL (bad) cholesterol, which is linked to heart attacks and strokes. Furthermore, it appears to slow down cartilage deterioration in osteoarthritis, a condition in which the joints are gradually worn down over time by wear and tear. On the nutrient front, this fruit provides vitamin C and potassium, both of which add to its heart health benefits.

Pomegranate may also have anti-viral and anti-bacterial properties, and has been shown to discourage the formation of dental plaque.

POMEGRANATE AND PEACH NECTAR

600ml/21fl oz/2⅓ cups
   pomegranate juice
2 peaches, pitted and chopped

Put the ingredients in a blender and whiz until smooth. Drink immediately.

kiwi fruit

Vitamins B3, B5, B6, C, E, beta-carotene, biotin, folate; calcium, copper, iodine, iron, magnesium, manganese, phosphorus, potassium, selenium, zinc; fibre; carbohydrate

GRILLED FRUIT KEBABS

3 kiwi fruit, peeled
½ pineapple, peeled
3 bananas
16 strawberries
6 tbsp pineapple juice
2 tbsp agave syrup or honey

Cut the kiwis, pineapple and bananas into 2.5-cm/1-in cubes. Thread alternate pieces of the cut-up fruit and strawberries onto wooden skewers. Combine the pineapple juice and agave syrup or honey in a bowl and use it to brush the kebabs. Then, place them under a grill for about 6 minutes, turning frequently.

Named after an indigenous New Zealand bird, kiwi fruit can combat the factors that cause heart disease and stroke.

Kiwi fruit have been found to have an anti-clotting effect, which is good news for people who are at high risk of heart disease and strokes. According to research, blood clotting was significantly reduced in those consuming two to three kiwi fruit a day. With further studies this fruit could possibly become a natural alternative to aspirin as a blood-thinning agent. In addition, kiwis act as a mild laxative, probably owing to their fibre content, and are a rich source of cell-protective antioxidants including vitamins C and E, beta-carotene and the phytochemical lutein, which helps to boost eye health.

papaya

Also known as paw paw, papaya can be eaten ripe as a succulent fresh fruit or cooked in curries and stews in its unripe green state.

Besides being a superb source of vitamin C and beta-carotene, which are important for the skin and immune system, papaya contains an enzyme called papain, which promotes the digestion of protein. Papain also soothes inflammation, so may be beneficial in easing joint pain from conditions such as arthritis and sports injuries. Used topically, papaya flesh is said to aid the healing of skin sores, while its edible seeds have been used to treat stomach aches and fungal infections.

NUTRIENTS
Vitamins B3, B5, C, beta-carotene, biotin, folate; calcium, iodine, iron, magnesium, manganese, phosphorus, potassium, selenium, zinc; fibre; carbohydrate

GET-UP-AND-GO JUICE

400ml/14fl oz/1½ cups apple juice
½ papaya, peeled and sliced
2 apricots, pitted and chopped
¼ avocado, peeled, pitted and chopped
250g/9oz/1 cup bio-yogurt
pinch of ground nutmeg

Put all the ingredients (except the nutmeg) in a blender and whiz until smooth. Serve sprinkled with nutmeg.

pineapple

NUTRIENTS
Vitamins B3, B5, C, E, K, beta-carotene, biotin, folate; calcium, copper, iron, magnesium, manganese, phosphorus, potassium, zinc; fibre; carbohydrate

Not only a delicious exotic fruit, pineapple has a special health asset in the form of bromelain, an enzyme that helps in the digestion of protein.

Research has shown that bromelain also works as an anti-inflammatory and is useful for the treatment of sprains, muscle injuries and post-operative inflammation by reducing pain and swelling. Pineapple is also a good source of manganese, an essential trace mineral needed for skin, bone and cartilage formation, and vitamin C, which mops up dangerous free radicals and enhances immune function.

POACHED PINEAPPLE

200ml/7fl oz/¾ cup grape juice
1 tbsp honey
½ pineapple, thickly sliced
juice of ½ orange

Put the grape juice and honey in a pan and bring to the boil. Add the pineapple and poach for 5 minutes. Place in a dish, squeeze over the orange juice and cook in a preheated oven at 200°C/400°F/Gas mark 6 for 10 minutes. Remove, return juices to the pan and reduce to a syrup. Pour over the pineapple and serve.

Sharon fruit (persimmon)

This tasty bright orange fruit can be eaten like an apple or pear, with or without the skin.

Sharon fruit is a type of persimmon, called "the food of the gods" by the ancient Greeks. It contains a broad range of nutrients including vitamin C, potassium, magnesium, calcium and fibre, all of which are vital for maintaining a healthy heart and keeping cholesterol levels in check. The fruit is also a good source of beta-carotene, which is required for the health of the skin and mucous membranes, and for night vision. Sharon fruit juice is believed to combat hangovers by lowering the density of alcohol in the blood.

NUTRIENTS
Vitamin C, beta-carotene, folate; calcium, iron, magnesium, phosphorus, potassium; fibre; carbohydrate

RAINBOW FRUIT SALAD WITH CHOPPED NUTS AND RAISINS

4 Sharon fruit
8 lychees, peeled and pitted
1 banana
8 fresh pitted dates
a handful of chopped hazelnuts
a handful of raisins
juice of 1 orange (or other fruit juice if preferred)

Chop the Sharon fruit, lychees, banana and dates and put them in a bowl along with the nuts and raisins. Pour the orange juice over the fruit, stir gently and serve.

oats

NUTRIENTS
Vitamins B1, B2, B3, B5, B6, E, K, biotin, folate; calcium, copper, iron, magnesium, manganese, phosphorus, potassium, selenium, silica, zinc; fibre; protein; complex carbohydrate

For blood sugar maintenance, sustained energy and staving off hunger, there's no better breakfast than a steaming bowl of cooked porridge oats.

The main feature in oats is a soluble fibre compound called beta-glucan, which decreases the glucose and insulin response after eating. This action makes it a beneficial food for diabetics or those with blood-sugar imbalances. Oats also enhance the immune system and significantly lower LDL (bad) cholesterol levels. In addition, they contain unique antioxidant compounds called avenanthramides, which prevent free-radical damage, thereby offering protection against cancer and heart disease.

RAISIN FLAPJACKS

300g/10½oz/3 cups porridge oats
100g/3½oz/¾ cup raisins
150g/5½oz unhydrogenated margarine
8 tbsp honey
6 tbsp fruit sugar
1 tbsp natural vanilla extract

Put the oats and raisins in a mixing bowl and set aside. Melt the margarine in a pan, add the remaining ingredients and stir. Pour onto the oats and mix well. Press into a non-stick baking tray, and cook in a preheated oven at 190°C/375°F/Gas mark 5 for 15–18 minutes.

barley

This glutinous grain has a chewy texture similar to pasta and is ideal eaten in soups and stews during the winter months to help warm the body.

An excellent source of slow-releasing carbohydrates, barley helps stabilize blood sugar levels, thereby preventing energy slumps and sugar cravings. It's also high in B-vitamins, which help to boost energy and combat stress, and a soluble fibre compound called beta-glucan that lowers raised cholesterol levels. Barley water, a drink made from the liquid in which barley has been boiled, is traditionally acclaimed for treating diarrhoea, fluid retention and cystitis.

NUTRIENTS
Vitamins B1, B2, B3, B5, B6, E, K, beta-carotene, folate; calcium, copper, iron, magnesium, manganese, phosphorus, potassium, silica, zinc; fibre; protein; complex carbohydrate

BARLEY AND VEGETABLE SOUP

55g/2oz pot barley, soaked overnight in cold water
2 tbsp olive oil
1 onion, chopped
1 clove garlic, crushed
2 celery sticks, chopped
1 tomato, chopped
1 tbsp paprika
55g/2oz green beans, chopped
1.5 litres/52fl oz/6 cups vegetable stock
1 tsp dried mixed herbs

Drain the barley and put it in a large pan. Add all the other ingredients, then bring to the boil and simmer, covered, for about 1 hour.

Choose "pot" barley rather than "pearl" barley, as it is less refined and therefore has more nutrients.

brown rice

NUTRIENTS
Vitamins B1, B3, B5, B6, E, K,
biotin, folate; calcium, copper,
iodine, iron, magnesium,
manganese, phosphorus,
potassium, selenium, zinc; fibre;
protein; complex carbohydrate

Providing more than one-fifth of the calories eaten
worldwide, rice, particularly in its unrefined form, is
one of the most nourishing food sources available.

According to the macrobiotic philosophy, brown rice is
considered to be the most balanced of all foods and those who
follow this dietary regime often eat it on a daily basis. When
consumed regularly it may help to ease depression, probably
due to its B-vitamin and magnesium content – nutrients needed
to calm and strengthen the nerves. It also helps stabilize blood
sugar levels and makes a wonderful convalescing food.

PILAU RICE

1 onion, finely chopped
1 tbsp olive oil
2 cardamom pods
5 cloves
½ cinnamon stick
pinch of saffron threads
200g/7oz brown basmati rice
**800ml/28fl oz/3 cups vegetable
    stock**
2 bay leaves

Sauté the onion in the oil until
soft. Add the spices and cook for
a further 2 minutes. Then add the
rice and stir until the grains are
coated in the oil before adding
the stock and bay leaves. Bring
to the boil, then simmer, covered,
for about 50 minutes or until the
rice is soft and all the liquid has
been absorbed.

TOXIN FIGHTER

Brown rice is a good source of insoluble fibre, helping to normalize and regulate bowel function, prevent constipation and remove toxins from the large intestine. Gamma oryzanol, a compound present in rice bran, may help to lower elevated cholesterol by increasing its excretion and reducing the absorption of cholesterol from food. Gamma oryzanol has also been found to aid in the relief of gastritis and other gastro-intestinal complaints.

GO FOR BROWN

The processing of wholegrain brown rice into white rice removes much of its B-vitamin and mineral content and all of its dietary fibre. So although brown rice takes a little longer to cook than white rice – about 45 minutes as opposed to 15 minutes – it's well worth the extra time.

COCONUT MILK RICE PUDDING

200g/7oz/1 cup short-grain brown rice
3 tbsp raisins
2 tbsp agave syrup
1 cinnamon stick
10 cardamom pods
400ml/14fl oz/1½ cups coconut milk
½ tsp natural vanilla extract
ground cinnamon

Put the rice, raisins, agave syrup, cinnamon stick and cardamom in a pan with 1 litre/35fl oz/4 cups water and bring to the boil. Simmer, covered, for 90 minutes until the water is absorbed. Add the coconut milk and vanilla. Cook for 5 minutes. Sprinkle with the ground cinnamon and serve.

millet

NUTRIENTS
Vitamins B1, B2, B3, B5, B6, E, K, folate; calcium, copper, iron, magnesium, manganese, phosphorus, potassium, selenium, silica, zinc; fibre; protein; complex carbohydrate

This small, round grain helps to feed the skin, hair and nails, and being free of gluten, it is well tolerated by most people.

Unlike most grains, millet is alkaline-forming, so it may help to neutralize acidic conditions in the body, such as rheumatism and arthritis. It's an excellent source of minerals, particularly calcium, magnesium and silica, all needed for healthy skin and strong hair and nails. In addition, magnesium plays an important role in hormonal balance, easing menstrual discomfort and water retention. As millet does not contain the gluten that wheat, barley and oats have, it is suitable for those with coeliac disease or other forms of gluten intolerance.

MILLET PATTIES

250g/9oz millet
1 tbsp olive oil
1 tbsp tomato purée
2 tbsp vegetable stock
1 tbsp tamari
2 tbsp unrefined sunflower oil

Bring 750ml/26fl oz/3 cups water to boil in a pan and simmer the millet, covered, for 45 minutes. Add the remaining ingredients (except the oil) and mix well. Form into patties, brush with oil and cook in a preheated oven at 190ºC/375ºF/Gas mark 5 for 40 minutes, turning them over halfway through.

quinoa

For centuries this grain-like seed sustained the Incas of South America and today it has superfood status thanks to its exceptional nutritional profile.

Unlike traditional cereals such as wheat and rice, quinoa contains all eight essential amino acids, making it a complete source of protein, normally found only in meat, fish, eggs, dairy and soya. This means that it's an ideal food for strict vegetarians or anyone who wants to boost their protein intake, such as athletes and those on high-protein weight-loss diets. Quinoa is also an excellent source of calcium and magnesium, which are needed for the bones, and iron, which prevents anaemia.

NUTRIENTS

Vitamins B1, B2, B3, B5, B6, E, folate; calcium, copper, iron, magnesium, manganese, phosphorus, potassium, zinc; fibre; protein; complex carbohydrate

QUINOA TABBOULEH

500ml/17fl oz/2 cups
   vegetable stock
250g/9oz/1¼ cups quinoa
3 tomatoes, chopped
½ cucumber, peeled and
   chopped
4 spring onions, trimmed and
   chopped
6 tbsp chopped parsley
2 cloves garlic, crushed
2 tbsp olive oil
2 tbsp lemon juice
sea salt and ground black
   pepper to taste

Bring the stock to boil in a pan and simmer the quinoa, covered, for 15 minutes. Transfer to a bowl, add the remaining ingredients and mix.

amaranth

A staple for the Aztec civilization of central Mexico, this tiny, nutritious grain is super-rich in protein, calcium and iron.

NUTRIENTS
Vitamins B1, B2, B3, B5, B6, C, E, folate; calcium, copper, iron, magnesium, phosphorus, potassium, zinc; fibre; protein; complex carbohydrate

Like quinoa, amaranth is a fantastic source of complete protein, along with fibre and complex carbohydrates. It is also high in calcium and contains more iron than most grains, so when eaten regularly can boost levels of this mineral. Several studies have shown that amaranth can reduce blood pressure and high cholesterol, as well as enhance the immune system. The active components responsible for these effects are thought to be plant stanols and squalene, important phytochemicals.

AMARANTH PANCAKES

100g/3½oz amaranth
1 tbsp arrowroot powder
1 tsp baking powder
pinch of sea salt
1 free-range egg
200ml/7fl oz soya milk
1 tbsp honey
2 tbsp unrefined sunflower oil

Grind the amaranth into a flour and put it in a bowl with the arrowroot powder, baking powder and salt. Add the egg, soya milk and honey and mix well. Pour a quarter of the batter into an oiled frying pan and cook on each side for 2 minutes. Repeat until all the batter is used up.

buckwheat

This unique-tasting grain blends well when mixed with blander grains and is marvellous for strengthening blood vessels and improving a sluggish circulation.

In spite of its name, buckwheat is not related to wheat and is suitable for those on a wheat- or gluten-free diet. Its main asset is its rich source of rutin, a bioflavonoid compound that helps strengthen weakened blood capillaries. In turn, this may improve circulatory problems such as capillary fragility, chilblains and high blood pressure. Buckwheat also appears to address glucose intolerance by aiding blood-sugar balance.

NUTRIENTS
Vitamins B1, B2, B3, B5, B6, E, K, folate; calcium, copper, iron, magnesium, manganese, phosphorus, potassium, selenium, zinc; fibre; protein; complex carbohydrate

Soba are a type of thin Japanese noodle, often made from buckwheat flour.

SOBA NOODLES IN PESTO SAUCE

4 tbsp olive oil
2 onions, chopped
2 cloves garlic, crushed
8 tomatoes, chopped
6 tbsp chopped basil
2 tsp dried basil
6 tbsp pine kernels
500g/1lb 2oz soba (buckwheat) noodles

Heat the oil in a pan and sauté the onion. Add the garlic and tomatoes and simmer, covered, for 20 minutes. Stir in the basil and pine kernels and cook for a few minutes. Put the mixture in a food processor and blend until creamy. Meanwhile, boil the soba noodles in water until *al dente* and serve with the pesto sauce.

aduki bean

NUTRIENTS

Vitamins B1, B3, B5, B6, E, beta-carotene, biotin, folate; calcium, copper, iodine, iron, magnesium, manganese, phosphorus, potassium, selenium, zinc; fibre; protein; complex carbohydrate

Try sprouting aduki beans as they are one of the easiest legumes to grow.

In Japan these small, red legumes are known as the "king of beans" and are the second most popular legume after the soya bean.

Containing more fibre and protein and less fat than most beans, adukis are the legumes of choice for anyone wanting to lose weight. Their high potassium content, which acts as a natural diuretic, adds to this weight-reducing effect by ridding the body of excess fluid. A drink made from the water in which aduki beans have been boiled is a traditional remedy for kidney and bladder complaints.

ADUKI BEAN CHILLI

100g/3½oz/½ cup aduki beans
1 onion, chopped
1 clove garlic, crushed
2 tbsp olive oil
400g/14oz tin chopped tomatoes
½ green chilli, deseeded and finely chopped
½ tsp chilli powder
1 tbsp tamari

Soak the beans overnight in cold water. Next day, drain, put in a pan with water and bring to the boil. Simmer, covered, for about 1 hour until soft. Drain and set aside. In another pan, gently fry the onion and garlic in the oil, add the remaining ingredients and the beans, and simmer, covered, for 25 minutes.

chickpea

Eaten as part of a balanced diet, chickpeas can help to keep high cholesterol in check and protect against heart disease.

High in both insoluble and soluble fibre, chickpeas not only maintain a healthy digestive system but significantly reduce both total and LDL (bad) cholesterol. Their role in heart health is also associated with their folate content, which lowers a compound called homocysteine in the blood, an excess of which is a risk factor for heart attack and stroke. Being rich in complex carbohydrates, chickpeas provide sustaining energy, while their substantial iron content may help to stave off anaemia.

NUTRIENTS
Vitamins B1, B2, B3, B5, B6, E, K, beta-carotene, biotin, folate; calcium, copper, iodine, iron, magnesium, manganese, phosphorus, potassium, selenium, zinc; fibre; protein; complex carbohydrate

CHICKPEA CURRY

150g/5½oz/⅔ cup chickpeas
1 onion, chopped
2 cloves garlic, crushed
2 tsp curry powder
2 tbsp olive oil
500ml/17fl oz/2 cups passata

Soak the chickpeas overnight in cold water. Next day, drain and put in a pan with water. Bring to the boil and simmer, covered, for 2 hours until soft. Drain and set aside. Then, sauté the onion, garlic and curry powder in the oil, stirring continually. Add the passata and cooked chickpeas and simmer, covered, for 25 minutes.

lentil

Lentils come in several varieties, including green, brown, red split and Puy, and are one of the best foods for balancing blood sugar levels.

With their low glycaemic index and complex carbohydrate content, lentils can prevent energy slumps by sustaining blood-sugar balance. They are also an excellent source of insoluble fibre, which helps to keep the bowel regular, as well as soluble fibre, which lowers high cholesterol levels. In addition to providing slow-releasing body fuel, lentils may help to combat fatigue by replenishing iron and B-vitamin stores.

NUTRIENTS

Vitamins B1, B2, B3, B5, B6, E, K, beta-carotene, biotin, folate; calcium, copper, iodine, iron, magnesium, manganese, phosphorus, potassium, selenium, zinc; fibre; protein; complex carbohydrate

RED LENTIL DHAL

2 tbsp olive oil
1 onion, chopped
2 cloves garlic, crushed
1 tsp ground mustard seeds
1 tsp ground cumin
½ tsp chilli powder
½ tsp turmeric
2 tomatoes, chopped
200g/7oz/¾ cup red lentils

Heat the oil in a pan and gently fry the onion until soft. Add the garlic, spices and tomatoes and simmer for a few minutes, stirring. Add the lentils and 500ml/17fl oz/2 cups water, bring to the boil and simmer, covered, for 20 minutes.

Lentils are best eaten with wholegrains where they fulfil the requirement of a complete protein.

soya bean

The health benefits of soya can be enjoyed in its many forms, such as tofu, tempeh, edamame, soya milk, miso, shoyu and tamari.

Unlike other legumes, soya is a source of complete protein, rivalling meat, fish and eggs. It is also rich in brain-boosting nutrients including essential fatty acids and lecithin, and contains isoflavones, a type of plant oestrogen, found to help balance oestrogen levels in the body. This makes soya useful in circumstances where oestrogen levels may be out of kilter, such as during the menopause. Soya isoflavones also appear to increase bone mass, offering protection against osteoporosis.

NUTRIENTS

Vitamins B1, B2, B3, B5, B6, E, K, beta-carotene, biotin, folate; calcium, copper, iodine, iron, magnesium, manganese, phosphorus, potassium, selenium, zinc; fibre; protein; complex carbohydrate; omega-3 and omega-6 essential fatty acids; lecithin

TOFU SCRAMBLER

500g/1lb 2oz tofu
2 tsp dried mixed herbs
2 tsp paprika
2 tsp ground mustard seeds
2 tsp tamari
2 tbsp chopped, flat-leaf parsley
3 tbsp olive oil
4 tbsp vegetable stock
1 onion, chopped

Mash the tofu in a bowl and mix in the dried herbs, paprika, mustard seeds, tamari and parsley. Set aside. Heat the oil and vegetable stock in a pan and gently fry the onion until soft. Add the tofu mixture and cook for about 8 minutes, stirring frequently.

almond

Crammed with goodness, these creamy-tasting nuts are ideal food for the brain and nervous system.

NUTRIENTS

Vitamins B1, B2, B3, B5, B6, E, biotin, folate; calcium, copper, iodine, iron, magnesium, manganese, phosphorus, potassium, selenium, zinc; fibre; protein; monounsaturated fats, omega-6 essential fatty acids

One of the most health-giving of all nuts, almonds are packed with nutrition. Their calcium and magnesium content aids bone-building and muscle function, while their high levels of vitamin E improve the skin, protect cells from free radicals and slow down the ageing process. Almonds also contain monounsaturated fats, which lower cholesterol levels. They are a rich source of protein, making them great for vegetarians. While high fat foods often cause weight gain, an almond-enriched diet has actually been found to help shed unwanted pounds.

RASPBERRY ALMOND TART

1 jar sugar-free raspberry jam
1 free-range egg, beaten
5 tbsp brown rice syrup
100g/3½oz/1 cup ground almonds
4 tbsp unrefined sunflower oil
5 tbsp rice milk
½ tsp natural vanilla extract
4 drops natural almond extract

Spread the jam into the base of an oven-proof dish. Put the remaining ingredients in a bowl, mix well and spoon the mixture evenly over the jam. Bake in a preheated oven at 190°C/375°F/Gas mark 5 for 40–45 minutes until golden and firm to the touch.

macadamia nut

High in monounsaturated fats, macadamias help to normalize blood cholesterol levels and improve overall heart health.

Including macadamia nuts regularly in the diet reduces LDL (bad) cholesterol levels, while increasing good HDL cholesterol. This effect is linked to the nut's high concentration of monounsaturated fats along with its plant sterol content, which inhibits the absorption of cholesterol from food. Macadamias are full of other nutrients, including potassium and magnesium, which help to regulate fluid balance, protein needed for growth and tissue repair, and cell-protective antioxidants such as vitamin E, selenium and a compound called epicatechin.

NUTRIENTS
Vitamins B1, B3, B5, B6, E, biotin; calcium, copper, iodine, iron, magnesium, manganese, phosphorus, potassium, selenium, zinc; fibre; protein; monounsaturated fats

MACADAMIA CRANBERRY CRUNCH

100g/3½oz/⅔ cup macadamia nuts
100g/3½oz/¾ cup dried cranberries
225g/8oz/1¾ cups rolled oats
2 tbsp brown rice syrup
2 tbsp unrefined sunflower oil
1 tbsp natural vanilla extract

Crush the nuts into small pieces in a food processor, then mix them with the other ingredients. Spread the mixture on a baking tray and toast in a preheated oven at 200°C/400°F/Gas mark 6 for 10 minutes, stirring halfway through. Use as a dessert topping.

walnut

NUTRIENTS

Vitamins B1, B2, B3, B5, B6, E, biotin; calcium, copper, iodine, iron, magnesium, manganese, phosphorus, potassium, selenium, zinc; fibre; protein; monounsaturated fats, omega-3 and omega-6 essential fatty acids

With their two-lobed appearance resembling a brain, it's no surprise that walnuts aid cognitive function and sharpen the memory.

Walnuts are not only a good source of heart-healthy monounsaturated fats, but also contain alpha-linolenic acid, an omega-3 essential fatty acid that makes them unique among nuts. Omega-3 fats provide cardiovascular protection and aid brain function; they're also anti-inflammatory and so are useful in the treatment of asthma, rheumatoid arthritis and skin disorders, such as eczema and psoriasis. In addition, walnuts contain the amino acid arginine, which helps to keep blood vessels flexible, and ellagic acid, an antioxidant that research has shown to have powerful anti-cancer properties.

WALNUT PESTO

a large handful of basil leaves
2 garlic cloves
20 walnuts
200ml/7fl oz/¾ cup olive oil

Put all the ingredients in a food processor and blend until creamy. Serve stirred into wholemeal pasta or noodles, or use as a dressing for steamed vegetables.

coconut

Nearly every part of this health-giving tropical nut is edible, including its flesh, oil and sap.

Although coconut is high in saturated fats, they're a different type to those found in meat and dairy and don't pose the same health risks. Known as medium chain fatty acids (MCFAs), they are easily digested and metabolized by the body, and are used as an energy source rather than being stored as fat. The coconut water – the liquid inside young coconuts – is known to be one of the most balanced electrolyte sources in nature, making a wonderful rehydration drink following intense exercise or when fluids and electrolytes have been lost through diarrhoea or fever.

NUTRIENTS
Vitamins B1, B2, B3, B5, B6, C, E, folate; calcium, copper, iodine, iron, magnesium, manganese, phosphorus, potassium, selenium, zinc; fibre; protein; carbohydrate; medium chain fatty acids

NON-ALCOHOLIC PIÑA COLADA

500ml/17fl oz/2 cups pineapple juice
200ml/7fl oz/¾ cup coconut water
small tin pineapple in fruit juice
55g/2oz creamed coconut

Put all the ingredients in a blender and whiz until smooth. Pour into a glass pitcher and stir well before serving with ice.

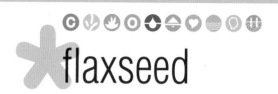

flaxseed

NUTRIENTS
Vitamins B1, B2, B3, B5, B6, E; calcium, copper, iron, magnesium, manganese, phosphorus, potassium, selenium, zinc; fibre; protein; omega-3 essential fatty acids

From preventing constipation to lowering high blood pressure and balancing hormones, flaxseed is truly a wonderfood.

Flaxseed (also called linseed) owes many of its healing properties to its omega-3 essential fatty acid content, which is converted in the body into hormone-like substances called prostaglandins. These are anti-inflammatory, and may benefit conditions such as asthma and arthritis. They also promote heart health by reducing cholesterol, blood pressure and plaque formation in the artery walls. Not only this, prostaglandins encourage weight loss by removing excess fluid from tissues and boosting metabolism, thereby helping to burn calories.

PEANUT FLAX BARS

100g/3½oz flaxseeds
150g/5½oz puffed rice cereal
5 tbsp crunchy peanut butter
5 tbsp brown rice syrup

Grind the flaxseeds in a nut grinder and put them in a large bowl. Add the puffed cereal, peanut butter and rice syrup, and mix well using your hands. Press the mixture very firmly into a non-stick baking tray and leave to stand for several hours before cutting into bars.

A GENTLE LAXATIVE
Another great feature of flaxseed is mucilage, a type of soluble fibre that lowers cholesterol, stabilizes blood sugar levels and alleviates constipation. Flaxseed's laxative effect is gentle, helping to keep intestinal contents moving smoothly along.

FIGHTS BREAST CANCER
The benefits of flaxseed do not stop there. This seed is also particularly rich in lignans, special compounds which are

converted by friendly bacteria in the gut into two hormone-like substances called enterolactone and enterodiol. These compounds have been found to offer protection against breast cancer, as well as helping to reduce the symptoms of hot flushes during the menopause.

Flaxseed also contains anti-viral, anti-bacterial and anti-fungal properties and helps to keep the skin looking youthful.

TROPICAL FLAX SHAKE

1 tbsp flaxseeds
600ml/21fl oz/2⅓ cups
**   pineapple juice**
200ml/7fl oz/¾ cup apple juice
2 kiwi fruit, peeled and
**   chopped**
2 passion fruit, halved

Grind the flaxseeds in a coffee grinder and put them in a blender along with the fruit juices and kiwi fruit. Scoop out the seeds from the passion fruit and add them to the juice mixture. Blend well and drink immediately.

pumpkin seed

NUTRIENTS
Vitamins B2, B3, B5, E, K,
beta-carotene; calcium, copper,
iron, magnesium, manganese,
phosphorus, potassium, zinc; fibre;
protein; omega-3 and omega-6
essential fatty acids

Exciting news for men: pumpkin seeds may offer
protection against prostate cancer.

Containing protein, vitamin E and zinc (needed to heal wounds,
maintain growth in children and boost immunity), pumpkin
seeds are a rich source of the essential fatty acids required
for hormone balance and healthy-looking skin. These seeds
are often recommended to men as a remedy for prostate
enlargement, as there are components in pumpkin seed oil
that interfere with prostate cell multiplication. The seeds also
make an effective dewormer and have been used to help to treat
roundworm, tapeworm and other intestinal parasites.

SEEDY MUFFIN CRUNCH

400g/14oz/3¼ cups flour
2 tsp baking powder
200g/7oz/1⅔ cups raisins
100g/3½oz pumpkin seeds
2 carrots, peeled and grated
4 free-range eggs, beaten
200ml/7fl oz/¾ cup maple syrup
200ml/7fl oz/¾ cup milk
**200ml/7fl oz/¾ cup unrefined
sunflower oil**

Combine the flour, baking
powder, raisins and seeds in a
bowl. Then, add the remaining
ingredients and mix well to form
a batter. Spoon the mixture into
an oiled muffin tray and bake in a
preheated oven at 180°C/350°F/
Gas mark 4 for 20 minutes or
until the muffins are a light
golden colour.

sesame seed

Exceptionally rich in calcium, sesame seeds are an excellent choice for nourishing the bones and teeth.

Often used to make tahini or sesame paste, these tiny seeds are packed with a broad range of minerals, including calcium, magnesium and manganese, along with generous helpings of protein and essential fatty acids. Containing 670mg of calcium per 100gm, they beat most foods, including whole milk, in the calcium stakes. In addition, sesame seeds contain a unique compound called sesamin, which has been shown to inhibit cholesterol absorption from food and prevent the development of high blood pressure.

NUTRIENTS

Vitamins B1, B2, B3, B5, B6, E, beta-carotene; calcium, copper, iodine, iron, magnesium, manganese, phosphorus, potassium, zinc; fibre; protein; omega-6 essential fatty acids

SESAME CHEWS

175g/6oz dried dates
55g/2oz chopped pecan nuts
2 tbsp tahini
2 tbsp peanut butter
4 tbsp sesame seeds

Put 250ml/9fl oz/1 cup water in a pan and simmer the dates, covered, for about 10 minutes until soft and all the liquid has evaporated. Mash the dates and mix together with the pecan nuts, tahini and peanut butter. Allow the mixture to stand for about 30 minutes so that it firms up, then form it into small balls and coat with sesame seeds.

hemp seed

This wholesome seed contains nature's most perfectly balanced source of essential fatty acids.

Hemp seeds have an excellent balance of essential fatty acids, and include omega-3 and omega-6 in the ideal ratio for good health. These fats are converted into hormone-like substances in the body called prostaglandins which govern many important functions including growth, vitality and mental well-being. Another important fat in hemp seeds is gamma-linolenic acid or GLA. People with eczema and other skin complaints are often deficient in this nutrient, so eating these seeds or taking hemp seed oil may be helpful in alleviating these conditions. In addition, hemp seeds contain complete protein, the quality of which is comparable to that found in meat, fish and eggs.

NUTRIENTS
Vitamins B1, B2, B6, C, E, beta-carotene; calcium, copper, iron, magnesium, manganese, phosphorus, potassium, zinc; fibre; protein; carbohydrate; omega-3 and omega-6 essential fatty acids, gamma-linolenic acid

---

HEMP SPRINKLE

3 tbsp pumpkin seeds
3 tbsp sunflower seeds
2 sun-dried tomatoes
½ tsp crushed dried chillies
6 tbsp shelled hemp seeds
1 tbsp sesame seeds
sea salt to taste (optional)

Grind the pumpkin seeds, sunflower seeds, sun-dried tomatoes and chillies. Put them in a bowl with the hemp seeds and sesame seeds and mix well. Add a little salt to taste if desired, and use as a sprinkle on salads and savouries.

alfalfa

Eaten sprouted, alfalfa is highly regarded for its amazing array of nutrients and enzymes.

Long popular among health-food enthusiasts, alfalfa sprouts are packed with enzymes and easily digestible nutrients, which are unleashed during the sprouting process. Besides being a storehouse of amino acids, vitamins and minerals, alfalfa contains several phytochemicals that can protect against disease. Canavanine, an amino acid analogue, exerts anti-carcinogenic activity, while the plant oestrogens found in this food help to balance hormones. Other compounds abundant in alfalfa sprouts include saponins, which reduce cholesterol by binding to it so that the body can excrete it, and chlorophyll, a powerful blood-builder and detoxifying agent.

NUTRIENTS

Vitamins B3, B5, C, K, beta-carotene, folate; calcium, iron, magnesium, phosphorus, potassium, zinc; protein; enzymes

TOFU, AVOCADO AND ALFALFA POCKETS

200g/7oz smoked tofu, sliced
4 wholemeal pitta breads
2 large handfuls of alfalfa
sprouts
2 avocados, peeled, stoned
and sliced
2 tomatoes, sliced
12 pitted black olives, chopped
2 tbsp tahini

Grill the tofu slices on both sides. Warm the pittas briefly in an oven, then cut them along the top and stuff with the tofu, alfalfa, avocados, tomatoes and olives. Put the tahini and 6 tbsp water in a bowl and mix well. Spoon it over the pitta filling and serve.

parsley

The world's most popular culinary herb, there's much more to parsley than its use as a garnish.

A rich source of cancer-fighting antioxidants, including vitamin C and the flavonoid luteolin, parsley has long been used to improve arthritic and rheumatic conditions. It helps to balance fluid levels in the body by increasing potassium status and encouraging the excretion of sodium and water. This makes parsley a natural herbal diuretic and may also help to control high blood pressure. When applied topically to the skin, the herb is said to relieve irritation caused by insect bites.

NUTRIENTS

Vitamins B1, B3, B5, C, E, K, beta-carotene, biotin, folate; calcium, iodine, iron, magnesium, manganese, phosphorus, potassium, selenium, zinc

---

PARSLEY PASTA SAUCE

2 tbsp olive oil
½ onion, chopped
1 garlic clove, crushed
1 tsp paprika
400ml/14fl oz/1⅔ cups
    passata
3 tbsp chopped parsley
sea salt and ground black
    pepper to taste

Heat the oil in a pan and gently fry the onion until soft. Add the garlic and paprika and continue to cook for 1 further minute, stirring. Add the passata and simmer, covered, for 20 minutes. Add the parsley and seasoning toward the end of cooking time. Serve over pasta.

Chewing on a parsley sprig after a meal can help to freshen the breath.

sage

Centuries-old theories about the healing properties of sage are now being proven by scientific research.

Not only does sage ease coughs and rheumatism, and strengthen the nervous system, but this versatile herb can also be added to gargles to relieve a sore throat and mouthwashes to combat gum inflammation. In Germany, sage has been approved for the treatment of mild gastro-intestinal complaints and excessive sweating. Thanks to its success in reducing perspiration, sage is now a popular remedy for preventing hot flushes during the menopause. The herb has also been found to boost memory by increasing levels of an important chemical messenger in the brain.

NUTRIENTS
Vitamins B3, B6, C, E, K, beta-carotene, biotin, folate; calcium, iron, magnesium, manganese, phosphorus, potassium, zinc

MASHED POTATOES WITH SAGE

4 large potatoes, peeled and diced
1 tbsp butter or unhydrogenated margarine
100g/3½oz soft goat's cheese
2 tbsp finely chopped sage
sea salt and ground black pepper

Steam the potatoes for about 20 minutes until soft. Transfer to a bowl, add the butter or margarine and mash well. Mix in the cheese and chopped sage, season to taste with salt and pepper, and serve.

garlic

NUTRIENTS
Vitamins B1, B3, B5, B6, C, biotin, folate; calcium, germanium, iodine, iron, magnesium, manganese, phosphorus, potassium, selenium, zinc; fibre

Garlic is a modern panacea, effective for fighting heart disease, cancer and a host of other afflictions.

Cultivated for more than 5,000 years, garlic has been appreciated for its healing properties since the days of the ancient Egyptians. As a folk remedy, it is used in many cultures to prevent colds and flu and in laboratory analysis it has been found to contain anti-bacterial, anti-viral and anti-fungal agents. A key active compound in garlic is allicin, which is produced from another compound, alliin, when fresh garlic is cut or crushed. Responsible for the bulb's pungent odour, this compound appears to be effective not only against common infections such as colds, flu and candidiasis (yeast infection), but also against more hazardous microbes, such as tuberculosis, as well as the superbug MRSA (methicillin-resistant *Staphylococcus aureus*).

GARLIC-INFUSED OLIVE OIL

250ml/9fl oz/1 cup extra virgin olive oil
8 garlic cloves
1 tsp crushed chillies

Buy a 250ml/9fl oz bottle of extra virgin olive oil and add the whole garlic cloves and chillies. Some of the oil may have to be removed before infusing so that it doesn't spill over. Secure the lid and leave in a cool, dark cupboard for several days to allow the flavours to mingle. Use as required for cooking or as a salad dressing.

HEALTHY BLOOD, LOW CHOLESTEROL

Garlic has many cardiovascular benefits and its regular consumption has been proven to lower both high blood pressure and cholesterol levels. It also inhibits blood-platelet stickiness, which is associated with the formation of blood clots, and heart attacks and strokes.

ANTI-CANCER WONDER HERB

Sulphur compounds in garlic, including allicin and diallyl sulphide, appear to protect the body against cancer-forming substances and may also halt the growth of cancer cells once they develop. Ajoene, which is produced from allicin may be useful in the treatment of skin cancer when applied topically. Other anti-cancer compounds in garlic include the powerful antioxidant minerals, germanium and selenium.

REFRIED BEANS

250g/9oz red kidney beans
3 tbsp olive oil
3 garlic cloves, crushed
1 tsp chilli powder
1 tsp ground cumin
1 tsp ground mustard seeds
1 tsp tamari

Soak the beans in cold water overnight. Next day, drain, then put in a pan and cover with water. Bring to the boil and simmer, covered, for about 2 hours. Drain and set aside. Put the remaining ingredients with 100ml/3½fl oz/⅓ cup water in another pan and sauté for a few minutes. Add the beans and mix well. Mash until creamy.

dill

NUTRIENTS
Vitamins B3, C, folate; calcium, iron, magnesium, phosphorus, potassium, zinc

Also known as dill weed, this herb is renowned as a treatment for digestive complaints in both adults and children.

Dill is effective for the relief of colic, gas and indigestion, and the active compound is thought to be an anti-spasmodic agent called carvone. Other components in dill have been found to indirectly neutralize cancer-forming substances, such as those in cigarette smoke and charcoal grill smoke (which may be ingested through barbecued food). Dill has also been studied for its ability to control the growth of bacteria. Taken as a tea, the herb is said to increase the production of breast milk.

> Fresh dill makes a tangy addition to pickles, salad dressings and fish dishes.

NEW POTATO SALAD WITH DILL

750g/1lb 10oz baby new potatoes
1 tbsp wholegrain mustard
2 tbsp olive oil
2 tbsp chopped dill
sea salt and ground black pepper

Cut the potatoes in half and steam them for about 15 minutes until cooked through. Put them in a large bowl, add all the other ingredients, mix well and serve.

mint

This herb has been treasured since ancient times for its culinary, medicinal and aromatic properties.

The essential oil in mint is known for its ability to improve food assimilation and relieve symptoms of irritable bowel syndrome, which it does by relaxing the smooth muscles in the intestinal tract. It has also been found to inhibit the growth of several types of bacteria, including *Helicobacter pylori* – now known to be the main cause of stomach and duodenal ulcers. In addition, mint contains rosmarinic acid, an anti-inflammatory compound that encourages cells to make substances that keep the airways open for easier breathing. This may make the herb useful for respiratory disorders such as asthma.

NUTRIENTS
Vitamins B1, B2, B3, B5, B6, C, E, beta-carotene, biotin, folate; calcium, magnesium, phosphorus, potassium

MINTY YOGURT DRESSING

300g/10½oz/1¼ cups bio-yogurt
2 tsp finely chopped fresh basil
1 tbsp finely chopped fresh mint
pinch of dried dill
ground black pepper to taste

Stir all the ingredients together in a bowl and chill. This dressing is especially good on cucumber or tomato-based salads or mixed into grated root vegetables.

mustard seed

NUTRIENTS
Vitamins B1, B2, B3, B5, B6, E, K, beta-carotene, biotin; calcium, copper, iodine, iron, magnesium, manganese, phosphorus, potassium, selenium, zinc

Available in three different colours – black, brown and yellow – ground mustard seeds make a flavoursome addition to a range of soups, casseroles and curries.

A relative of broccoli and cabbage, mustard seeds contain phytochemicals unique to this food family known as glucosinolates. These compounds have been well-studied for their ability to stop the growth of existing cancer cells and to prevent new cancer cells from forming. This spice is also an excellent source of the mineral selenium, an important antioxidant with anti-inflammatory properties. Taken crushed in a little warm water, mustard seeds are believed to purify the blood and have a mild laxative effect.

PAN-FRIED CAULIFLOWER WITH BEETROOT AND MUSTARD SEEDS

2 tbsp olive oil
2 tbsp mustard seeds
½ tsp paprika
2 raw beetroot, peeled and cut into thin strips
1 cauliflower, broken into small florets
4 tbsp vegetable stock

Heat the oil in a lidded pan, add the mustard seeds, cover and gently fry until they pop. Add the paprika and vegetables and cook for 2 minutes. Add the stock and simmer for about 8 minutes, stirring frequently.

turmeric

This bright yellow spice has powerful properties which help to alleviate pain and inflammation.

A main spice ingredient in curries, the key active constituent in turmeric is curcumin which has been found to have a number of therapeutic actions. It reduces pain and inflammation and is commonly employed in the treatment of rheumatoid arthritis and other forms of joint pain. In fact, it may even be more effective in this area than conventional anti-inflammatory drugs. Turmeric also contains antioxidant properties, is liver-protective and appears to prevent platelet stickiness, which may guard against heart disease and strokes.

NUTRIENTS

Vitamins B3, C, E, K, folate; calcium, iron, magnesium, manganese, phosphorus, potassium, selenium, zinc

THAI CURRY SAUCE

400ml/14fl oz/1½ cups coconut milk
2 green chillies, deseeded and chopped
2 garlic cloves
2 tsp grated fresh ginger root
2 shallots, chopped
1 tbsp olive oil
1 lemongrass stalk, peeled
1 tsp turmeric
2 tbsp chopped coriander

Put the coconut milk, chillies, garlic and ginger in a blender and whiz. Heat the oil, add the shallots and gently fry until soft. Add the coconut mixture and the remaining ingredients. Bring to the boil and simmer for 5 minutes. Serve with rice.

ginger

NUTRIENTS
Vitamins B3, C, E, folate; calcium, iron, magnesium, phosphorus, potassium, selenium, zinc

With its soothing, pain-relieving and anti-inflammatory properties, ginger is invaluable as a medicinal food.

Widely employed in African, Chinese and Indian cuisines, ginger can be cooked in food to add a zingy flavour or made into a medicinal tea. But the use of ginger extends well beyond its role in the kitchen. Historically, it has been utilized for its effect on the digestive tract where it calms the stomach, dispels gas, eases nausea and aids the absorption of nutrients.

Ginger is extremely effective as a remedy for motion or sea sickness, reducing all associated symptoms including dizziness and vomiting. It is also helpful in relieving morning sickness during pregnancy, but unlike drug-based anti-emetics that can cause harmful side effects, ginger is safe to take.

CREAMY GINGER DRESSING

4 tbsp tahini
2 tsp grated fresh ginger root
1 garlic clove
1 tsp tamari
2 tsp brown rice syrup

Put all the ingredients in a blender with 5 tbsp water and whiz until creamy. Serve stirred into noodles or as a salad dressing.

COMBATS ARTHRITIS

A proven treatment for osteoarthritis and rheumatoid arthritis, ginger helps to reduce pain and swelling in the joints, and improves mobility when taken on a regular basis. Its ability to work in this way has been attributed to its antioxidant properties and its potent anti-inflammatory compounds called gingerols, which suppress the substances that trigger joint inflammation.

HEART PROTECTION

Ginger supports heart health by preventing blood platelets from sticking together and lowering cholesterol levels, thereby offering protection against heart attacks and strokes. It also stimulates the circulation and is excellent for alleviating coughs and fever caused by colds or flu.

RASPBERRY GINGER WHIP

2 tsp grated fresh ginger root
200g/7oz raspberries
450g/1lb crème fraîche
a handful of crystallized
ginger, chopped

Put the ginger root and raspberries in a food processor and blend. Add the mixture to the crème fraîche and stir. Serve chilled in individual dessert glasses, sprinkled with a few pieces of chopped crystallized ginger.

cinnamon

NUTRIENTS
Vitamins B2, B3, B5, B6, E, K, beta-carotene, biotin; calcium, copper, iodine, iron, magnesium, manganese, phosphorus, potassium, selenium, zinc

Highly prized since antiquity, cinnamon was regarded as a gift fit for kings and it is said that wars were even fought over it.

Used traditionally for its warming qualities, cinnamon may help to ward off colds and improve the circulatory system. It contains anti-bacterial and anti-fungal properties that have been found to inhibit organisms such as *Candida albicans*, a yeast responsible for causing candidiasis and thrush. In addition, research has shown that compounds in cinnamon lower blood sugar levels, which is thought to make it a promising remedy for type 2 diabetes.

CINNAMON CREAM

250g/9oz tofu
10 tbsp apple juice
3 tbsp brown rice syrup
3 tbsp unrefined sunflower oil
½ tsp ground cinnamon

Put all the ingredients in a food processor and blend until smooth and creamy. Use as a substitute for dairy cream on desserts.

Purchase Ceylon cinnamon as its flavour is more refined than the Indonesian variety.

087

cardamom

Sweet and aromatic, cardamom is not only a wonderful flavouring agent but is also an antidote for a plethora of health complaints.

Cardamom can be used whole or ground to flavour both sweet and savoury dishes, and it is often made into a soothing tea. The spice stimulates the appetite and the flow of saliva, making it helpful during convalesence when the desire for food may be lacking. It can also be used to treat gum infections, sore throats and bad breath – in India it was often employed as a gargle for this purpose. In traditional Chinese medicine, cardamom is valued as a remedy for treating stomach upsets, flatulence and other problems of the digestive system.

NUTRIENTS
Vitamins B3, C; calcium, iron, magnesium, manganese, phosphorus, potassium, zinc

HOT CARDAMOM COCOA

8 cardamom pods
1 litre/35fl oz/4 cups soya milk
2 tbsp chocolate drink powder
2 tbsp agave syrup
1 tsp natural vanilla extract
50g/1¾oz dark chocolate, grated
1 tsp ground cardamom

Bruise the cardamom pods with the flat edge of a knife and put them in a saucepan. Add the soya milk, chocolate powder, agave syrup and vanilla extract and bring it to the boil very slowly, stirring frequently. Strain into four mugs, sprinkle with the grated chocolate and ground cardamom, and serve immediately.

egg

Extremely versatile, eggs pack a punch on the nutritional front and are an incredible brain food.

Eggs are highly nutritious, supplying an excellent source of complete protein important for tissue repair, along with vitamins A, B12 and D, which are lacking in many foods. They also contain omega-3 fats and a B-vitamin called choline, both of which are required for normal brain function, and lutein, which can help to reduce the risk of eye disease. The nutritional value of eggs has been found to vary, with the free-range variety containing more vitamins and good fats, and less cholesterol than eggs laid by battery hens.

NUTRIENTS

Vitamins A, B2, B3, B5, B6, B12, D, E, biotin, folate; calcium, chromium, copper, iodine, iron, magnesium, manganese, phosphorus, potassium, selenium, sodium, zinc; protein; omega-3 fatty acids

---

POTATO FRITTATA

450g/1lb potatoes, peeled and diced
1 tbsp olive oil
4 free-range eggs, beaten
1 tbsp soya sauce
5 tbsp chopped parsley
ground black pepper to taste

Steam the potatoes for 15 minutes, then transfer to the pan oiled with the olive oil. Mix together the remaining ingredients and pour them over the potatoes. Cook gently for 3–4 minutes. Once the underside is done, place under a grill and cook until golden and set.

bio-yogurt

With its rich probiotic content, bio-yogurt helps to keep the digestive system in good shape by boosting the population of friendly gut bacteria.

Produced by the fermentation of milk, bio-yogurt contains "live" bacteria including lactobacillus and bifido, which help to maintain levels of beneficial bacteria in the intestinal tract. Through this action, bio-yogurt can help to prevent constipation and alleviate the bloating, gas and vaginal thrush often caused by an overgrowth of candida yeast. It can also avert antibiotic-related diarrhoea and keep invading organisms in check, in addition to supporting the immune system.

NUTRIENTS

Vitamins A, B2, B3, B5, B12, C, D, biotin, folate; calcium, iodine, iron, magnesium, phosphorus, potassium, selenium, zinc; protein

AMBROSIA FRUIT SALAD

2 tbsp flaked almonds
2 tbsp flaked coconut
small tin crushed pineapple, drained
1 banana, chopped
200g/7oz cherries, pitted
6 tbsp bio-yogurt
2 tbsp pure maple syrup
1 tsp ground cinnamon
½ tsp ground nutmeg

Toast the almonds and coconut in a dry pan for a few minutes then transfer to a bowl and leave to cool. Add the fruit and yogurt and mix together so that all the ingredients are well combined. Spoon into individual dessert bowls, top with maple syrup, cinnamon and nutmeg and serve.

salmon

Packed with health-giving essential fatty acids, salmon is also an excellent source of protein.

NUTRIENTS
Vitamins A, B1, B2, B3, B5, B6, B12, D, E, biotin, folate; calcium, iodine, iron, magnesium, phosphorus, potassium, selenium, zinc; protein; omega-3 fatty acids

Falling into the oily fish category, salmon contains omega-3 fats in the form of eicosapentaenoic acid (EPA) and docosahexaenoic acid (DHA). These fatty acids have been found to have numerous health benefits including lowering cholesterol and high blood pressure, easing the symptoms of asthma, rheumatoid arthritis and depression, and improving skin conditions such as eczema and psoriasis. DHA also boosts intelligence in children. In addition, salmon is a valuable source of B-vitamins and the mineral selenium, while wild salmon is rich in astaxanthin, one of the most potent antioxidants ever discovered.

BAKED SALMON WITH CAPER AND TOMATO DRESSING

4 salmon fillets
1 tbsp capers, chopped
4 cherry tomatoes, chopped
1 shallot, chopped
1 tbsp lemon juice
2 tbsp olive oil

Put each salmon fillet on a piece of greased foil. Mix the remaining ingredients in a bowl and spoon over the fillets. Fold up the foil to form parcels. Place them on a baking tray and bake in a preheated oven at 200°C/400°F/Gas mark 6 for 10–12 minutes until the fish is cooked. Serve.

turkey

Being one of the leanest forms of animal protein, this traditional festive food makes a healthier alternative to other meat and poultry.

Relatively low in fat, turkey is a superb source of protein, which the body needs for tissue growth and repair. It also contains several B-vitamins, crucial for normal metabolism and the health of the nervous system. Turkey is a rich source of anaemia-preventing iron and the powerful anti-cancer mineral selenium, which is usually found only in small amounts in many foods. As with all meat and poultry, buying organic is the best choice, because it is likely to be lower in calories and to contain a better ratio of good to bad fats.

NUTRIENTS
Vitamins B2, B3, B5, B6, B12, D, biotin, folate; calcium, iodine, iron, magnesium, phosphorus, potassium, selenium, zinc; protein

TURKEY AND PEPPER CHIMICHANGAS

2 turkey breasts, diced
1 red onion, chopped
1 red pepper, cut into strips
1 tbsp unrefined sunflower oil
6 tbsp shop-bought salsa
4 large flour tortillas
a handful of grated cheese

Stir-fry the turkey, onion and pepper in the oil for 5–6 minutes. Add the salsa and heat through. Warm the tortillas in the oven and place the mixture in the centre of each. Roll them up and place them seam-side down on a baking tray and top with cheese. Bake in a preheated oven at 180°C/350°F/ Gas mark 4 for 10–12 minutes.

apple cider vinegar

NUTRIENTS
Vitamins B1, B2, B6, C, E, beta-carotene; calcium, chlorine, fluorine, iron, magnesium, manganese, phosphorus, potassium, selenium, silica, sulphur, zinc

It is thought that Hippocrates, the father of modern medicine, used apple cider vinegar as a healing elixir to treat his patients.

Made from the fermented juice of pressed apples, 90 different beneficial substances have been discovered in apple cider vinegar, including carbolic acids, enzymes and trace minerals, which help to balance the body's acid–alkaline levels. Through its alkalizing effect, it is reported to alleviate a number of complaints, such as arthritis, rheumatism, headaches, heartburn and muscle cramps. The vinegar is also used as a weight-loss enhancer, which it achieves by improving fat digestion, metabolism and liver detoxification.

FRENCH DRESSING

3 tbsp apple cider vinegar
6 tbsp olive oil
4 tbsp unrefined sunflower oil
½ tsp wholegrain mustard
½ tsp paprika
½ tsp dried mixed herbs
1 garlic clove, crushed
sea salt and ground black pepper

Place all the ingredients in a clean screwtop jar, seal, put on the lid and shake vigorously. Store in the fridge for up to a week and use on salads as required.

miso

There are several types of miso available, but the darker varieties are a wise choice, as they are richer in protein and essential fatty acids.

A naturally fermented paste made from soya beans, sea salt and koji (a yeast mould), miso is a tasty replacement for salt and adds flavour to soups, sauces and casseroles. It's an excellent source of protein, minerals and B-vitamins, and contains soya isoflavones – plant oestrogens associated with reducing the symptoms of the menopause and the risk of osteoporosis and breast cancer. It also boasts dipicolonic acid, a compound that binds to toxic metals in the body, such as mercury and lead, and removes them via the intestinal tract.

NUTRIENTS
Vitamins B1, B2, B3, B5, B6, K, beta-carotene, folate; calcium, copper, iron, magnesium, manganese, phosphorus, potassium, selenium, sodium, zinc; protein; omega-3 and omega-6 essential fatty acids

MISO SOUP

1 tbsp sesame oil
2 spring onions, trimmed and chopped
100g/3½oz smoked tofu, cut into small cubes
1 carrot, peeled and cut into matchsticks
1 tbsp miso

Heat the oil in a pan, add the onion, tofu and carrot and gently fry for a few minutes until soft. Add 800ml/28fl oz/3¼ cups water and the miso, and simmer for 5 minutes. Serve with brown rice, noodles or wholegrain bread.

umeboshi plum

This popular Japanese plum possesses a range of restorative qualities, including helping the body to recover more quickly from the effects of alcohol.

NUTRIENTS
Vitamins B1, B2, B3; calcium, iron, phosphorus, potassium, sodium; fibre

Pickled in sea salt, these tangy, tart plums are often puréed and eaten with rice. Traditionally, umeboshi plums have been used for aiding digestion and combating fatigue, actions which are thought to be linked to their alkalizing effect and ability to reduce lactic acid, a build-up of which can lead to exhaustion. In addition, the fruit's pyric acid content stimulates the function of the liver and kidneys to dissolve and expel toxins from the body, thereby enhancing the breakdown of alcohol and making these exotic plums a good remedy for hangovers.

UMEBOSHI VINAIGRETTE

8 tbsp sesame oil
4 tbsp rice vinegar
1 tbsp umeboshi paste
1 tsp brown rice syrup

Put all the ingredients in a screwtop jar, seal and shake vigorously. Keep refrigerated and use on salads as required.

kuzu

In addition to being a natural thickening agent, kuzu is a wonderful remedy for colds, headaches and all kinds of digestive upsets.

Prepared from the root of a Japanese vine, kuzu's main role in the kitchen is as a thickening agent, where it adds body to soups, stews and sauces. Besides its culinary uses, kuzu has been valued as a medicine in China and Japan for hundreds of years. It's long been a traditional remedy for warding off colds and soothing irritated mucous membranes, thereby easing intestinal pain, cramp and diarrhoea. It is also used as an alternative to aspirin for headaches, and works by altering the chemicals in the brain called neurotransmitters.

NUTRIENTS
Calcium, iron, phosphorus, potassium; carbohydrate

VEGETARIAN GRAVY

2 tbsp kuzu
1 tbsp olive oil
1 tsp miso
½ tsp vegetable bouillon powder
1 tsp tamari or shoyu

Put the kuzu and 4 tbsp cold water in a bowl and mix until dissolved. Set aside. Put the remaining ingredients and 500ml/17fl oz/2 cups water in a pan and bring to the boil. Reduce the heat and stir in the dissolved kuzu. Continue to stir over a low heat until the liquid begins to thicken. Serve hot or cold.

carob

For anyone wishing to avoid chocolate, carob provides a tasty, caffeine-free alternative that is lower in fat and calories.

NUTRIENTS
Vitamins B1, B2, B3, B6, C, E, folate, beta-carotene; calcium, copper, iron, magnesium, manganese, phosphorus, potassium, selenium, silica, zinc; fibre; protein; carbohydrate

Derived from the pods of the carob tree, carob has a similar flavour to chocolate and is often used as a substitute in cakes, biscuits and desserts. The tannins in carob powder have an astringent effect on the intestines, making it useful for treating diarrhoea in both adults and children. It has also shown some promise in reducing high cholesterol, thanks to its significant dietary fibre content.

FROZEN CAROB BANANAS

4 bananas
4 wooden sticks
200g/7oz bar of carob
55g/2oz crushed nuts

Peel the bananas and cut them in half. Insert a wooden stick into the flat end of each banana half, put them on a lined tray and freeze them for about 2 hours. Melt the carob in a double boiler, then dip each banana into the carob and coat well. Finally, roll them in nuts and refreeze. Serve frozen.

Unlike chocolate, which is toxic to most animals, carob-based treats are considered safe for pets.

dark chocolate

Craved more than any other food in the world, chocolate – mainly the dark variety – delivers several health benefits.

Chocolate lovers can delight in the knowledge that their favourite treat is good for them. Studies have shown that dark chocolate, which has a high cocoa content, contains epicatechin and gallic acid, antioxidants with heart-protective properties. These compounds may promote anti-cancer activity, too. Chocolate also possesses phenylethylamine, an amphetamine-like compound that acts as a natural mood enhancer, and theobromine, which is a mild stimulant. To reap the benefits of dark chocolate, it should be eaten regularly in small amounts.

NUTRIENTS
Vitamins B3, B5, E, beta-carotene, biotin, folate; calcium, copper, iron, iodine, magnesium, manganese, phosphorus, potassium, selenium, zinc; fibre; protein; carbohydrate

CHOCOLATE MARZIPAN

175g/6oz/1⅔ cups ground almonds
4 tbsp brown rice syrup
1 tbsp natural almond extract
100g/3½oz dark chocolate

Mix together the ground almonds, brown rice syrup and almond extract to form a thick paste. Using your hands, roll the mixture into small balls (should make about 14) and set aside. Break the chocolate into pieces and melt it in a double boiler. Dip the balls in the melted chocolate, place them on a lined tray and leave to set.

honey

Besides being a natural sweetener, honey has many wonderful properties, including substances that speed up wound healing and fight superbugs.

Produced by bees from flower nectar, honey is the most natural of all sweeteners and is a viable replacement for sugar. As an energy source, it enhances sports performance by providing a welcome boost both during and after exercise. No wonder honey is considered a general pick-me-up!

ANTIOXIDANT POWER

Containing small amounts of vitamins, minerals and amino acids, honey appears to improve the status of protective antioxidants in the blood when consumed on a regular basis. In addition, a spoonful of honey with lemon in hot water can also soothe a sore throat and help to ease the symptoms of coughs and colds.

SUPERBUG SUPER-FIGHTER

There is a specific type of New Zealand honey called Manuka, which has been found to have powerful antibiotic properties. These inhibit the growth of bacteria, including *Helicobacter pylori*, which is associated with causing most stomach and

HONEY ALMOND CUP

500ml/17fl oz/2 cups rice milk
200g/7oz/1⅓ cups almonds
2 tbsp clear honey
1 tbsp natural vanilla extract

Put the rice milk and almonds in a blender with 300ml/10½fl oz/1¼ cups water and mix well. Pour the liquid through a sieve into a glass pitcher. Stir in the honey and vanilla extract, then chill in the fridge. Serve.

duodenal ulcers. The anti-bacterial activity of this honey is also proving to be an effective weapon in combating superbugs, such as MRSA (Methicillin-resistant *Staphylococcus aureus*), strains of which have become particularly resistant to conventional antibiotic treatment.

Manuka honey can also be used topically in the healing of skin ulcers, wounds, boils and burns, where it reduces inflammation and promotes tissue regeneration. Moreover, because it also has potent anti-fungal properties, this special honey has been used effectively to treat athlete's foot and other fungal infections.

BANANA, HONEY AND NUT BAGELS

4 wholegrain bagels
6 tbsp crunchy peanut butter
4 bananas, chopped
4 tsp clear honey
½ tsp ground cinnamon

Cut the bagels in half and spread each side with peanut butter. Set aside. Mash the bananas and mix them with the honey and cinnamon, then spoon the mixture on top of the peanut butter. Grill the bagels for a few minutes topping side up and serve immediately.

blackstrap molasses

This thick, dark, sticky syrup helps nourish red blood cells and boost flagging energy levels.

A by-product of the sugar cane refining process, this nutritious sweetener imparts a robust, bitter-sweet flavour and can be added to biscuits, tomato sauces and home-made baked beans. Often recommended as a remedy for anaemia, just one dessert spoon of blackstrap molasses provides around a quarter of an adult's daily iron needs. It is a good source of other minerals, such as calcium, which is needed for bone maintenance, and manganese, which plays a role in nerve health. It can also be taken as a supplement to improve general nutrient status.

NUTRIENTS

Vitamins B1, B2, B3, B5, B6, folate; calcium, chromium, copper, iron, magnesium, manganese, phosphorus, potassium, selenium, zinc; carbohydrate

BOSTON BAKED BEANS

200g/7oz haricot beans
1 tsp garlic powder
1 tsp ground mustard seeds
2 tbsp olive oil
1 tsp dried oregano
2 tbsp tomato purée
3 bay leaves
2 tsp blackstrap molasses

Soak the beans overnight in cold water. Next day, drain, and put in a pan with water. Bring to the boil and simmer for 2 hours until soft. Drain and set aside. Sauté the garlic and mustard seeds in the oil. Add 500ml/ 17fl oz/2 cups water and the remaining ingredients including the beans, and simmer, covered, for 15 minutes.

xylitol

Xylitol looks and tastes just like white sugar, but rather than encouraging dental caries, it has been found actually to reduce tooth decay.

Extracted from the wood fibre of birch trees, xylitol is a type of carbohydrate that can be used spoon for spoon instead of sugar in drinks, desserts and baking. However, because it has a very low glycaemic index, it's suitable for diabetics and those with poor blood sugar balance. Unlike other sweeteners, xylitol inhibits the development of tooth decay by reducing the secretion of plaque acids, especially in people who use xylitol-containing chewing gum or toothpaste on a regular basis.

NUTRIENTS
Carbohydrate

CAROB BROWNIES

100g/3½oz unhydrogenated
margarine
100g/3½oz/½ cup xylitol
200g/7oz/1 cup rice flour
4 tbsp carob powder
2 tbsp arrowroot powder
1 tsp baking powder
a handful of chopped walnuts
200ml/7fl oz/¾ cup rice milk
1 tbsp natural vanilla extract

Cream together the margarine and xylitol, then add the rice flour, carob, arrowroot and baking powder, and mix. Add the remaining ingredients and mix well. Spoon into an oiled baking tray, spread evenly and bake in a preheated oven at 180°C/350°F/Gas mark 4 for 30 minutes.

ailments directory

ANAEMIA

watercress (p.25), Jerusalem artichoke (p.35), kombu (p.44), nori (p.46), dulse (p.48), quinoa (p.79), amaranth (p.80), chickpea (p.83), lentil (p.84), alfalfa (p.95), turkey (p.111), blackstrap molasses (p.120).

ARTHRITIS

celery (p.16), radicchio (p.23), olive and olive oil (p.29), kombu (p.44), cherry (p.54), raspberry (p.61), goji berry (p.62), açai berry (p.63), pomegranate (p.68), papaya (p.71), pineapple (p.72), millet (p.78), walnut (p.88), flaxseed (p.90), parsley (p.96), turmeric (p.103), ginger (p.104), salmon (p.110), apple cider vinegar (p.112), kuzu (p.115).

ASTHMA

fennel (p.15), radicchio (p.23), sweet potato (p.39), butternut squash (p.42), nori (p.46), raspberry (p.61), açai berry (p.63), walnut (p.88), flaxseed (p.90), mint (p.101), salmon (p.110).

CANCER

cucumber (p.12), tomato (p.13), red pepper (p.14), fennel (p.15), celery (p.16), leek (p.18), aubergine (p.19), asparagus (p.20), globe artichoke (p.21), lettuce (p.22), radicchio (p.23), spinach (p.24), watercress (p.25), shiitake mushroom (p.27), olive and olive oil (p.29), cabbage (p.30), broccoli (p.32), carrot (p.33), beetroot (p.34), Jerusalem artichoke (p.35), mooli (p.36), potato (p.38), sweet potato (p.39), yam (p.40), butternut squash (p.42), kombu (p.44), hijiki (p.49), apple (p.50), grape (p.53), prune (p.58), blueberry (p.59), cranberry (p.60), raspberry (p.61), goji berry (p.62), açai berry (p.63), tangerine (p.64), grapefruit (p.65), lemon (p.66), pomegranate (p.68), oats (p.74), almond (p.86), walnut (p.88), flaxseed (p.90), alfalfa (p.95), garlic (p.98), dill (p.100), mustard seed (p.102), turmeric (p.103), turkey (p.111), miso (p.113), dark chocolate (p.117).

CANDIDIASIS

garlic (p.98), ginger (p.104), cinnamon (p.106), bio-yogurt (p.109).

COMMON COLD

tomato (p.13), red pepper (p.14), aubergine (p.19), lettuce (p.22), watercress (p.25), shiitake mushroom (p.27), broccoli (p.32), carrot (p.33), potato (p.38), sweet potato (p.39), horseradish (p.41), nori (p.46), blueberry (p.59), raspberry (p.61), goji berry (p.62), tangerine (p.64), grapefruit (p.65), lemon (p.66), guava (p.67), pomegranate (p.68), garlic (p.98), ginger (p.104), cinnamon (p.106), kuzu (p.115), honey (p.118).

CONSTIPATION

globe artichoke (p.21), okra (p.26), cabbage (p.30), beetroot (p.34), agar-agar (p.43), apple (p.50), pear (p.51), grape (p.53), fig (p.57), prune (p.58), raspberry (p.61), açai berry (p.63), grapefruit (p.65), kiwi fruit (p.70), oats (p.74), barley (p.75), brown rice (p.76), millet (p.78), quinoa (p.79), amaranth (p.80), buckwheat (p.81), chickpea (p.83), lentil (p.84), flaxseed (p.90), mustard seed (p.102), bio-yogurt (p.109).

COUGHS

carrot (p.33), horseradish (p.41), lemon (p.66), sage (p.97), ginger (p.104), honey (p.118).

DEPRESSION (MILD)

banana (p.52), goji berry (p.62), brown rice (p.76), almond (p.86), walnut (p.88), egg (p.108), salmon (p.110), dark chocolate (p.117).

DIABETES

leek (p.18), okra (p.26), shiitake mushroom (p.27), avocado (p.28), Jerusalem artichoke (p.35), sweet potato (p.39), yam (p.40), hijiki (p.49), blueberry (p.59), guava (p.67), oats (p.74), barley (p.75), brown rice (p.76), millet (p.78), quinoa (p.79), amaranth (p.80), buckwheat (p.81), chickpea (p.83), lentil (p.84), cinnamon (p.106), turkey (p.111), xylitol (p.121).

DIARRHOEA

banana (p.52), date (p.56), guava (p.67), barley (p.75), coconut (p.89), bio-yogurt (p.109), kuzu (p.115), carob (p.116).

EYE DISEASE

asparagus (p.20), spinach (p.24), watercress (p.25), broccoli (p.32), carrot (p.33), nori (p.46), blueberry (p.59), goji berry (p.62), kiwi fruit (p.70), egg (p.108).

FATIGUE

cucumber (p.12), celery (p.16), shiitake mushroom (p.27),

eddo (p.37), potato (p.38), sweet potato (p.39), yam (p.40), butternut squash (p.42), banana (p.52), date (p.56), prune (p.58), oats (p.74), barley (p.75), brown rice (p.76), millet (p.78), quinoa (p.79), amaranth (p.80), buckwheat (p.81), chickpea (p.83), lentil (p.84), coconut (p.89), umeboshi plum (p.114), dark chocolate (p.117), honey (p.118), blackstrap molasses (p.120).

GUM INFLAMMATION

cranberry (p.60), pomegranate (p.68), sage (p.97), cardamom (p.107), bio-yogurt (p.109), xylitol (p.121).

HEART DISEASE

tomato (p.13), fennel (p.15), celery (p.16), leek (p.18), asparagus (p.20), globe artichoke (p.21), spinach (p.24), watercress (p.25), okra (p.26), shiitake mushroom (p.27), avocado (p.28), olive and olive oil (p.29), carrot (p.33), agar-agar (p.43), wakame (p.47), hijiki (p.49), apple (p.50), pear (p.51), grape (p.53), blueberry (p.59), raspberry (p.61), açai berry (p.63), tangerine (p.64), grapefruit (p.65), pomegranate (p.68), kiwi fruit (p.70), Sharon fruit (p.73), oats (p.74), barley (p.75), brown rice (p.76), millet (p.78), quinoa (p.79), amaranth (p.80), buckwheat (p.81), chickpea (p.83), lentil (p.84), soya bean (p.85), almond (p.86), macadamia nut (p.87), walnut (p.88), flaxseed (p.90), sesame seed (p.93), hemp seed (p.94), garlic (p.98), turmeric (p.103), ginger (p.104), salmon (p.110), carob (p.116), dark chocolate (p.117).

HIGH BLOOD PRESSURE

celery (p.16), leek (p.18), shiitake mushroom (p.27), olive and olive oil (p.29), potato (p.38), kombu (p.44), wakame (p.47), dulse (p.48), banana (p.52), grape (p.53), açai berry (p.63), pomegranate (p.68), amaranth (p.80), buckwheat (p.81), flaxseed (p.90), sesame seed (p.93), hemp seed (p.94), parsley (p.96), garlic (p.98), salmon (p.110).

INDIGESTION

globe artichoke (p.21), radicchio (p.23), mooli (p.36), horseradish (p.41), kombu (p.44), papaya (p.71), pineapple (p.72), mint (p.101), ginger (p.104), bio-yogurt (p.109), apple cider vinegar (p.112), umeboshi plum (p.114).

INFLUENZA

red pepper (p.14), aubergine

(p.19), lettuce (p.22), watercress (p.25), shiitake mushroom (p.27), broccoli (p.32), horseradish (p.41), blueberry (p.59), raspberry (p.61), goji berry(p.62), tangerine (p.64), grapefruit (p.65), lemon (p.66), pomegranate (p.68), garlic (p.98), ginger (p.104), honey (p.118).

IRRITABLE BOWEL SYNDROME

fennel (p.15), globe artichoke (p.21), okra (p.26), brown rice (p.76), millet (p.78), flaxseed (p.90), dill (p.100), mint (p.101), ginger (p.104), cardamom (p.107), bio-yogurt (p.109), kuzu (p.115).

MENOPAUSE

fennel (p.15), soya bean (p.85), flaxseed (p.90), alfalfa (p.95), sage (p.97), miso (p.113).

OSTEOPOROSIS

spinach (p.24), watercress (p.25), broccoli (p.32), kombu (p.44), nori (p.46), wakame (p.47), hijiki (p.49), fig (p.57), pineapple (p.72), quinoa (p.79), amaranth (p.80), soya bean (p.85), sesame seed (p.93), bio-yogurt (p.109), miso (p.113).

RHEUMATISM

celery (p.16), kombu (p.44), cherry (p.54), millet (p.78), parsley (p.96), sage (p.97), ginger (p.104), apple cider vinegar (p.112).

SKIN COMPLAINTS

cucumber (p.12), tomato (p.13), avocado (p.28), olive and olive oil (p.29), carrot (p.33), wakame (p.47), açai berry (p.63), guava (p.67), papaya (p.71), walnut (p.88), flaxseed (p.90), pumpkin

seed (p.92), hemp seed (p.94), salmon (p.110).

UNDER-ACTIVE THYROID

kombu (p.44), nori (p.46), wakame (p.47), dulse (p.48), hijiki (p.49).

URINARY TRACT INFECTIONS

horseradish (p.41), blueberry (p.59), cranberry (p.60), raspberry (p.61), barley (p.75), aduki bean (p.82), garlic (p.98).

WATER RETENTION

cucumber (p.12), tomato (p.13), celery (p.16), asparagus (p.20), lettuce (p.22), Jerusalem artichoke (p.35), eddo (p.37), potato (p.38), sweet potato (p.39), yam (p.40), horseradish (p.41), banana (p.52), date (p.56), barley (p.75), aduki bean (p.82), parsley (p.96).

glossary

Alginic acid A polysaccharide in various sea vegetables that has the ability to remove heavy metals from the body.

Allicin A compound in garlic that has potent anti-bacterial and anti-fungal activities.

Anthocyanins Colourful pigments in various fruit and vegetables that are powerful antioxidants.

Antioxidants Compounds abundant in fruit and vegetables that inhibit the effects of damaging free radicals.

Beta-cryptoxanthin A carotenoid compound with antioxidant activity found in winter squash, papaya and watermelon.

Beta-glucan Soluble fibre with many health-giving attributes found in barley and oats.

Beta-sitosterol A phytosterol compound found in many natural foods that lowers cholesterol.

Bromelain An enzyme in pineapple that aids protein digestion and has anti-inflammatory effects.

Caffeic acid An antioxidant compound in many fruits, vegetables and herbs.

Calcium pectate A type of fibre that adds crispness to fruits and vegetables, and has powerful cholesterol-lowering properties.

Carotenoids Coloured pigments in various fruit and vegetables, which function as antioxidants. Some of them are converted in the body into vitamin A.

Carvone A natural anti-spasmodic agent found in the oils of dill and caraway seed.

Diallyl sulphide A sulphur compound with anti-cancer activity found in garlic.

Diindolylmethane A compound found in broccoli and other cruciferous vegetables, which

has anti-cancer, anti-viral and anti-bacterial properties.

Electrolyte A substance containing free ions, such as sodium, potassium, calcium, magnesium and chloride.

Ellagic acid A polyphenol antioxidant with anti-cancer properties found in many fruit and vegetables.

Flavonoids An umbrella term for a class of antioxidants found in many natural foods.

Free radicals Highly reactive molecules linked to causing degenerative diseases and the ageing process.

Fucoidan A polysaccharide in various sea vegetables that appears to destroy cancer cells.

Glucosinolates Compounds that have anti-cancer activity, found in broccoli, cabbage, Brussels sprouts, mustard seeds and other Brassicaceae.

Hesperidin A flavonoid antioxidant in citrus fruit that has anti-cancer and heart-protective properties.

Homocysteine An amino acid in the blood, high levels of which are linked to an increased risk of heart disease and stroke.

Inulin A type of carbohydrate that does not elevate blood sugar levels and so may help in the management of diabetes.

Isoflavones Phyto-oestrogen compounds found in soya and other foods that have oestrogen-like actions in the body.

Kaempferol A flavonoid antioxidant in fennel, broccoli, grapefruit and other plant-derived sources.

Limonene A cancer-fighting compound in citrus fruit.

Lutein An antioxidant carotenoid associated with eye health.

Lycopene An antioxidant carotenoid found in red foods, such as tomatoes, that has anti-cancer properties.

Melatonin A potent antioxidant produced by the body's pineal gland that helps to regulate sleep patterns.

Pectin A type of soluble fibre in fruit and vegetables that lowers cholesterol levels.

Phenylethylamine A natural mood-enhancing chemical found in chocolate.

Phytochemical Natural plant compounds abundant in fruit and vegetables that possess antioxidant activity.

Phytosterols Plant compounds that help to lower high cholesterol levels.

Proanthocyanidins A class of flavonoids with antioxidant activity found in various berries. They also help with skin maintenance and strengthen blood vessels.

Pterostilbene A compound present in blueberries and grapes, which has anti-cancer and cholesterol-lowering properties and is thought to reduce cognitive decline.

Quercetin An anti-inflammatory flavonoid that is particularly abundant in capers, apples and onions.

Resveratrol An antioxidant found in grapes and blueberries that has anti-cancer, anti-inflammatory and anti-viral properties.

Rutin A flavonoid antioxidant that helps to strengthen the blood vessels.

Squalene A compound found in amaranth seed, rice bran, wheat germ and olives that can help to reduce high blood pressure and elevated cholesterol levels.

Sulforaphane A cancer-fighting compound that can be obtained by eating cruciferous vegetables such as broccoli, Brussels sprouts and cabbage.

Tangeritin A cholesterol-lowering antioxidant found in tangerines and other citrus fruit.

Zeaxanthin An antioxidant carotenoid associated with eye health.

index